AF773026

W. W. Fleischhacker and D. J. Brooks (eds.)

Neuropsychopharmacology

Journal of Neural Transmission
Supplement 64

SpringerWienNewYork

Prof. Dr. W. Wolfgang Fleischhacker
Department of Biological Psychiatry
Innsbruck University Clinics
Anichstrasse 35
A-6020 Innsbruck, Austria

Prof. Dr. David J. Brooks
MRC Cyclotron Unit
Hammersmith Hospital
Du Cane Road
London W12 0NN, United Kingdom

Typesetting: Best-Set Typesetter Ltd., Hong Kong
Printing: A. Holzhausen`s Nfg., A-1140 Wien

Printed on acid-free and chlorine-free bleached paper

SPIN: 10904503

CIP data applied for

With 17 Figures

ISSN 0303-6995
ISBN 3-211-83902-X (soft cover) Springer-Verlag Wien New York
ISBN 3-211-83903-8 (hard cover) Springer-Verlag Wien New York

Preface

The 5th Neuropsychiatry Symposium of the European Institute of Healthcare was devoted to neuropsychopharmacology. As in previous meetings, we sought to choose topics that bridge the gap between basic neuroscience and the clinical fields of neurology and psychiatry. Consequently, the proceedings published in this supplement cover a lot of ground. Late breaking data on various neuromodulator and neurotransmitter systems and their implications for the treatment of a number of disorders are reviewed. Jean-Charles Schwartz and colleagues set the stage with their paper on constitutive receptor activity, using the histamine H3-receptor to illustrate the point. The role of neuropeptides and neurotrophins in psychiatric disorders is then reviewed by Florian Holsboer, while Bill Deakin elucidates the role of serotonin, discovered 50 years ago in the brain, in select psychiatric syndromes. New pharmacological developments in the treatment of migraine, Parkinson's disease and schizophrenia are then presented by Hans Christoph Diener, Eduardo Tolosa and Wolfgang Fleischhacker. In the end David Nutt and colleagues provide future directions in substance dependence research, linking the role of various transmitter systems with findings from neuroimaging studies. In summary, there is no doubt that progress in the field of neuropsychopharmacology is exciting and the prospects of true advances in the treatment of brain disorders are very promising.

Innsbruck/London, April 2003

W. W. Fleischhacker
D. Brooks

Contents

Listed in Current Contents/Life Sciences

J Neural Transm (2003) [Suppl] 64: 1–16

Therapeutic implications of constitutive activity of receptors: the example of the histamine H_3 receptor

J.-C. Schwartz[1], **S. Morisset**[1], **A. Rouleau**[1], **X. Ligneau**[2], **F. Gbahou**[1], **J. Tardivel-Lacombe**[1], **H. Stark**[3], **W. Schunack**[3], **C. R. Ganellin**[4], and **J. M. Arrang**[1]

[1] Unité de Neurobiologie et Pharmacologie Moléculaire (U. 573) INSERM, Centre Paul Broca, and
[2] Laboratoire Bioprojet, Paris, France
[3] Institut für Pharmazie, Freie Universität Berlin, Berlin, Federal Republic of Germany
[4] University College London, London, United Kingdom

Summary. Some G-protein-coupled receptors display constitutive activity, that is spontaneous activity in the absence of agonist: a proportion of the receptor population adopts a conformation that can bind and activate G proteins. Whereas this was mainly shown to occur with recombinant or pathologically mutated receptors, the physiological relevance of the process has remained debated. We have adressed this question in the case of the histamine H_3 receptor, a presynaptic inhibitory receptor regulating histamine release in brain. Having identified a neutral antagonist and inverse agonists with variable intrinsic activity, we show that the native H_3 receptor in brain displays high constitutive activity in vitro and, in vivo, controls the release of endogenous histamine. This implies that inverse agonists with high intrinsic activity should be preferred for therapeutic application as "cognitive enhancers" in several psychiatric disorders.

Introduction

The concept of constitutive activity arose from observations that receptors in certain biological systems were activated in the absence of any ligand. One correlate of this concept is the existence of a novel pharmacological entity the inverse agonists, i.e. a class of drugs able to reduce the activity of receptors in such systems. Hence, in addition to agonists able to activate receptors in a partial or full manner and antagonists which block the effect of agonists, the recently introduced class of inverse agonists has received a large attention during the last decade (Lefkowitz et al., 1993; Kenakin, 1997; Milligan and Bond, 1997; Leurs et al., 1998; Strange, 2002).

Although the first example of constitutive activity was described at the benzodiazepine, site of the GABA receptor, many examples were later shown at heptahelical receptors coupled to G proteins. In these receptors, constitutive activity is assumed to correspond to a pre-coupling to the G protein in the absence of agonist. Since this class of receptors is the target of a large fraction of drugs currently used in therapeutics, the concept could be of obvious practical importance. In agreement a large fraction of drugs previously known as antagonists have been recognized to act in fact as inverse agonists on relevant systems. Furthermore it has proved difficult to identify true neutral antagonists, i.e. drugs able to block the effects of either the agonists or the antagonists.

Many models were proposed to account for this "revised" pharmacology which have all in common to assume the existence of at least two conformers of the receptor, one inactive (uncoupled) and the other active (coupled). In this scheme i) the agonist is a drug binding preferentially to and stabilizing the active conformer R*; ii) the inverse agonist binds preferentially to and stabilizing the inactive conformer R; iii) the neutral antagonist is a drug displaying equal affinity for R and R*, a condition obviously difficult to fulfill which explains the low number of such compounds that could be recognized.

One important consequence of the concept is that several inverse agonists may display distinct intrinsic activity (like agonists themselves) which differs from the previously held idea that antagonists were all equivalent in terms of efficacy. Hence receptor ligands should be considered as triggering a continuum of effects from partial agonists to neutral antagonists and up to full inverse agonists.

It should be noted, however, that constitutive activity of receptors was described in most cases in artificial systems so that the physiological relevance of the process has remained debated. Normal recombinant receptors display clear constitutive activity when they are expressed at high density in transfected cells: by increasing the stoechiometry of receptor proteins in the membrane the chances for interacting with neighbouring G proteins is obviously enhanced.

Another circumstance is site-directed mutagenesis taking place in regions of the receptor governing the interaction with G proteins, first shown among adrenergic receptors mutated at the level of the third intracellular loop (Lefkowitz et al., 1993). Agonist-independent activity of heptahelical receptors consequent to a pathological mutation was shown to be the molecular basis for a series of human diseases, e.g. familial male precocious puberty (LH-receptor mutation), familial hyperthyroidism (TSH-receptor mutation) or hyperfunctional thyroid adenomas (TSH-receptor mutation).

Nevertheless the idea that constitutive activity may be operant at native non-mutated receptors, expressed at normal levels in tissues, has remained debated. We have undertaken to explore this idea in the case of the histamine H_3 receptor and to assess its implications for the design of ligands to be used in the treatment of CNS disorders.

The histamine H_3 receptor, a presynaptic inhibitory heptahelical receptor

The third histamine receptor subtype (H_3R) was identified by purely pharmacological approaches, i.e. using drugs to characterize a biological response. In 1983, Arrang et al. shown that endogenous histamine release from depolarized cerebral neurons was modulated by an autoreceptor displaying a pharmacological profile distinct from those of the H_1 and H_2 receptors that were the only ones known at this time (Arrang et al., 1983). Four years later, through a collaboration of the same group with two university groups of pharmacochemists, the first potent and highly selective ligands (agonists, partial agonists and antagonists) and radioligands were designed, clearly establishing the pharmacological identity of the receptor (Arrang et al., 1987). Whereas the belonging of the H_3R to the superfamily of G protein-coupled heptahelical receptors was soon demonstrated by the observation that H_3R binding of a radioligand agonist was modulated by guanylnucleotides, efforts to clone the receptor cDNA by homology or expression remained unsuccessful. In 1999, Lovenberg et al. identified within a private database of expressed sequence tags (ESTs) and using an α_2-adrenergic receptor sequence as query an EST displaying ~35% homology with the latter protein. The full sequence had clearly an organization of aminergic heptahelical receptor and, since the H_3R was one of the very last members of the superfamily defined pharmacologically but not yet cloned, Lovenberg et al. having expressed the orphan receptor in an heterologous cell system tested the hypothesis that it was the H_3R. Both radioligand binding data and responses to selective agonists clearly confirmed that they had cloned the human H_3R.

Starting from the sequence of the human H_3R, we screened a cDNA library from rat striatum and isolated two full-length cDNAs encoding 445- and 413-aminoacid sequences (Fig. 1) that we termed H_{3L} and H_{3S} in analogy with the corresponding H_3R variants in the guinea pig brain (Tardivel-Lacombe et al., 2000). The existence of these variants results from alternative splicing at the level of the pre-mRNA corresponding to the mid-portion of the third intracellular loop of the H_3R. The pharmacology of the two isoforms, as studied in transfected CHO cells, does not seem to differ markedly.

Constitutive activity of recombinant H_3 receptors

After cloning the rat H_3R, we noticed that the carboxy terminus of i3 has a stretch of eight amino acids strikingly similar to the corresponding sequence of a mutated human β_2-adrenergic receptor in which the mutation confers a constitutive activity (CAM hβ_2-AR in Fig. 1) that is absent in the native receptor (Samama et al., 1993). Thus, among these eight amino acids, six (five in the mouse) are identical in the rat H_3 receptor and in the mutated β_2-adrenergic receptor, whereas the other two amino acids are conserved. Furthermore, this region is also critical for constitutive activity in other native or mutated heptahelical receptors.

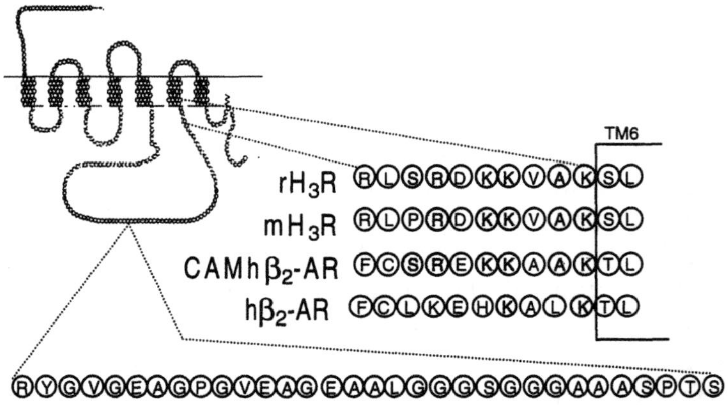

Fig. 1. Two rat H_3-receptor isoforms and their expression in rat brain regions. Putative seven-transmembrane topography of H_{3S} and H_{3L} alternatively spliced variants differing by a 32-aminoacid insertion in the i3 loop. This loop C-terminal sequence is also compared to that of the mouse (mH_3R), the native human β_2-adrenergic receptor ($h\beta_2$-AR) and a constitutively active mutant (CAM $h\beta_2$-AR) (Samama et al., 1993) (reproduced with permission from Morisset et al., 2000)

We have, therefore, assessed the constitutive activity of the H_{3L} and H_{3S} isoforms, i.e., $H_{3(445)}$ and $H_{3(413)}$ respectively, expressed in CHO cells at low, medium and high densities, i.e., 30–80, 300–500 and ~1,000 fmol/mg protein as determined by [^{125}I]iodoproxyfan assay (Ligneau et al., 1994), respectively. The coupling changes associated with receptor expression were evaluated in two signalling pathways activated by histamine and involving G_i/G_o-proteins, i.e., adenylyl cyclase inhibition and phospholipase A_2 activation. In both pathways, constitutive activity of both the H_{3L} and H_{3S} receptors was clearly evidenced. In agreement, [^{3}H]arachidonic acid ([^{3}H]AA) release evoked by the Ca^{2+}-ionophore A23187 was enhanced (Fig. 2) whereas forskolin-induced cAMP accumulation was reduced (in both cases in total absence of histamine) when the receptor density was enhanced. These changes were largely reversed in the presence of thioperamide, a compound so far considered as the prototypical H_3-receptor antagonist (Arrang et al., 1987), but appearing here, as predicted by binding data (Clark and Hill, 1995), as an extremely potent inverse agonist.

Constitutive activity was slightly more pronounced with the H_{3L} isoform: there was already a tendency to spontaneous activity and a response to thioperamide at low expression levels of H_{3L} (effects that became significant at 80 fmol/mg protein, not shown), and, at intermediate levels, changes were more marked than with the H_{3S} isoform (Fig. 2).

These observations could be repeated using cells expressing the human H_3R instead of the rat H_3R (Rouleau et al., 2002). Constitutive activity was assessed at similar H_3R densities (200–300 fmol/mg protein) and was found of similar amplitude in the two species when phospholipase D activation was monitored and ciproxifan (Ligneau et al., 1998) used as an inverse agonist. However using another test, the binding of [^{35}S]GTPγ[S], the human receptor displayed clearcut but somewhat lower constitutive activity (Fig. 3).

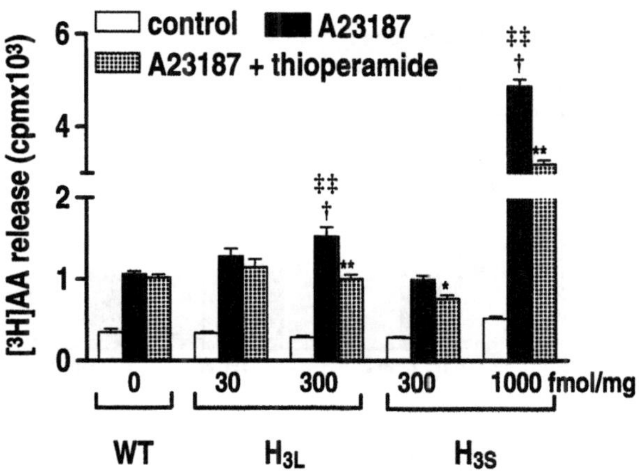

Fig. 2. Constitutive activity and pharmacology of H_{3S} or H_{3L} receptors expressed in CHO cells. Effects of thioperamide on [^{3}H]AA release evoked by 2 μM A23187 in CHO cells expressing various densities of the two H_3-receptor isoforms. Means ± SEM of 3–10 determinations in an experiment that was replicated with similar data. *P < 0.05, **P < 0.001 vs A23187 alone; †P < 0.001 vs wild-type cells; ‡P < 0.01; ‡‡P < 0.001 vs CHO(H_{3S}) cells expressing 300 fmol/mg protein (ANOVA followed by Newman-Keuls test) (reproduced with permission from Morisset et al., 2000)

We used the same test system to evaluate the effects of varying the level of hH_3R density in CHO cells on responses to imetit, a selective agonist, and ciproxifan acting as an inverse agonist (Fig. 4).

As previously shown for other GPCRs (Chidiac et al., 1994; Pozvek et al., 1997; Claeysen et al., 1999; Newman-Tancredi et al., 2000), we reported that constitutive activity of the recombinant rH_3R was positively correlated to receptor density and was favoured upon overexpression (Morisset et al., 2000). This observation, attributable to an increased receptor/G-protein stoichiometry (Kenakin, 1997), could be made with the hH_3R. Indeed, the increment of [^{35}S]GTPγ[S] binding due to the transfected receptor was 4-fold greater (~20 and 5 fmol mg^{-1} protein, respectively) at ~700 fmol mg^{-1} protein versus ~300 fmol mg^{-1} protein of hH_3R. The extended ternary complex model which describes two receptor states whereby the active state interacts with G proteins (Samama et al., 1993), predicts that the same maximal response that is produced by an agonist should be observed constitutively with high receptor expression levels. However, the increase in [^{35}S]GTPγ[S] binding (i.e. constitutive activity) observed at the highest densities of hH_3R was still substantially lower than the increase in binding induced by imetit (i.e. the agonist-induced maximal response), suggesting that the amount of receptor may be limiting for constitutive activity of the hH_3R. Consistent with this proposal, the increment in [^{35}S]GTPγ[S] binding observed at a receptor density of 1 pmol mg^{-1} protein was not significantly higher than that observed at ~700 fmol mg^{-1} protein. However, it was already significant at moderate densities (<500 fmol mg^{-1} protein), i.e. consistent with natural cellular levels of receptors, indicating that the threshold expression level for constitutive activity, which varies with the different types of receptors (Chen et al., 2000), is rather small for the hH_3R.

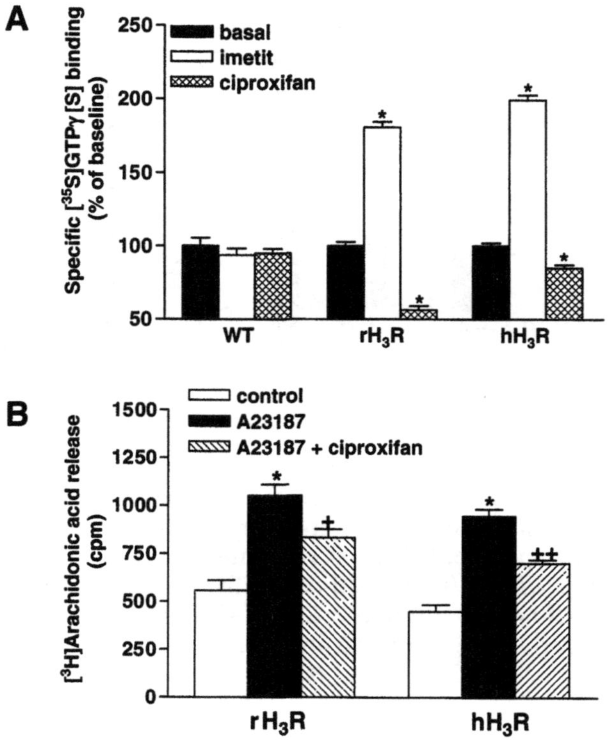

Fig. 3. Effects of H_3-receptor ligands on two responses mediated by the recombinant rat and human H_3 receptors. **A** Effects of H_3-receptor ligands on specific [^{35}S]GTPγ[S] binding. Membranes of wild-type CHO cells (WT) or cells expressing ~200–300 fmol mg^{-1} protein of rat (rH_3R) or human (hH_3R) receptors were incubated with 0.1 nM [^{35}S]GTPγ[S] and, when required, 1 μM imetit or ciproxifan. Data represent means ± SEM of 11–16 determinations from two separate experiments. *$P < 0.001$ vs the corresponding basal. **B** Effect of ciproxifan on A23187-evoked [^{3}H]arachidonic acid release. After incubation with 0.5 μCi of [^{3}H]arachidonic acid, CHO(rH_3R) and CHO(hH_3R) cells were incubated with 2 μM A23187 and, when required, 1 μM ciproxifan. Data are means ± SEM of 11–32 determinations from three to four experiments. *$P < 0.001$ vs the corresponding control; $^+P < 0.01$, $^{++}P < 0.001$ vs A23187

This suggests that constitutive activity of the native H^3R may be present not only in rodent brain (Morisset et al., 2000) but also in human brain.

Identification of a neutral antagonist: proxyfan

The above observations suggested that constitutive H_3-receptor activity was likely to occur in brain where the H_{3L} isoform predominates and where the density of [^{125}I]iodoproxyfan binding sites (Ligneau et al., 1994) is presumably more than 500 fmol/mg protein in cells expressing the H_3 receptor (assuming that these cells represent less than 20% of the total). To assess this possibility, we needed to identify ligands displaying well-defined agonist, inverse agonist, and neutral antagonist properties in cell lines and, then to determine the effects of these probes at the native cerebral receptor. Neutral antagonists are

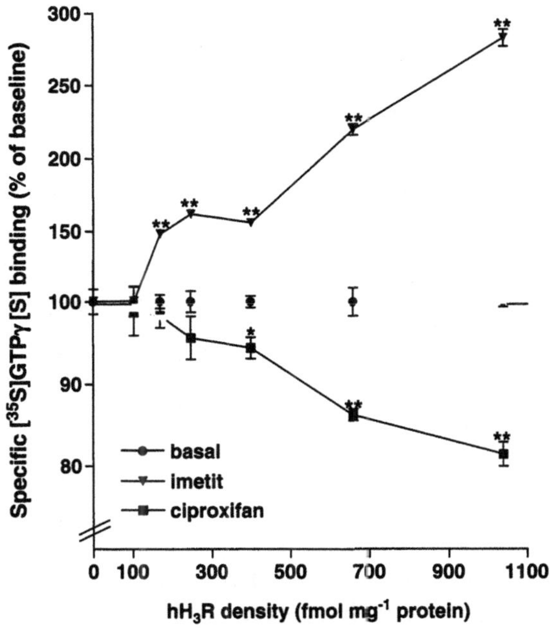

Fig. 4. Effects of H_3-receptor ligands on specific [^{35}S]GTPγ[S] binding to membranes from CHO cells expressing various densities of the human H_3 receptor (hH_3R). Membranes of CHO(hH_3R) cells expressing increasing densities of the human receptor (up to 1 pmol mg^{-1} protein) were incubated with 0.1 nM [^{35}S]GTPγ[S] and, when required, imetit or ciproxifan (1 μM). hH_3R densities were determined using [^{125}I]iodoproxyfan assay. Data represent means ± SEM of 8–14 determinations from two separate experiments. *$P < 0.01$ and **$P < 0.001$ vs the corresponding basal

not easily identified because, theoretically, they correspond to ligands displaying equal affinity for the active and inactive receptor conformations, a condition obviously difficult to achieve (Costa et al., 1992; Milligan et al., 1995). In agreement, a large number of tested antagonists (defined by their ability to block the histamine response at the autoreceptor inhibiting [^{3}H]histamine release from synaptosomes) behaved as potent inverse agonists: they decreased [^{3}H]arachidonic acid (AA) release from CHO cells at concentrations up to two orders of magnitude less than those required to antagonize histamine at the H_3 autoreceptor in synaptosomes. This included FUB 465 (ethyl-3-(1H-imidazol-4-yl)propyl ether), an antagonist with only micromolar affinity at the synaptosomal autoreceptor and exerting inverse agonist activity with an EC_{50} of ~10 nM in CHO(H_3) cells (Fig. 5).

After testing a large variety of compounds, we identified proxyfan (3-(1H-imidazol-4-yl)propyl-phenylmethyl ether) as a potent (Ki ~10 nM) neutral antagonist: i) it inhibited the effects of histamine at the synaptosomal H_3 autoreceptor, ii) in CHO(H_3) cells with moderate expression, it inhibited those of the agonist imetit as well as those of the inverse agonists ciproxifan and FUB 465, without affecting [^{3}H]AA release alone, even at a 10 μM concentration (Fig. 5). As expected, however, the pharmacological profile of proxyfan depended on the test system, i.e. on the equilibrium between the

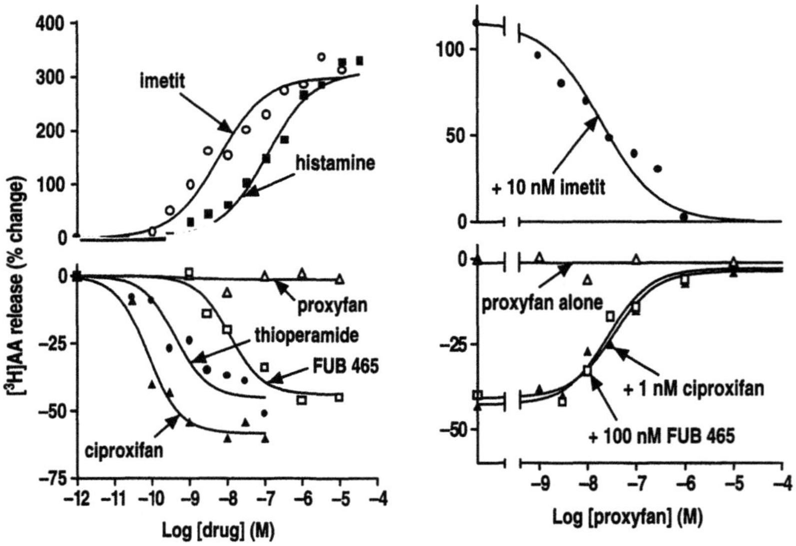

Fig. 5. Effects of H_3-receptor ligands on A23187-evoked [^{3}H]AA release from CHO cells expressing the H_{3S} receptor (500 fmol/mg protein). Release (cpm/well) evoked by A23187 was of 1281 ± 59 (over a basal value of 584 ± 28) and data are expressed in percent change of this value. Proxyfan (3-(1H-imidazol-4-yl)propyl-phenylmethyl ether) antagonized the effects of imetit, an agonist, and ciproxifan or FUB 465 (ethyl-3-(1H-imidazol-4-yl ether), two inverse agonists (reproduced with permission from Morisset et al., 2000)

active and inactive conformations of the receptor and/or the stoichiometric ratio of the receptor to the various G proteins: proxyfan displayed partial inverse agonism on [^{3}H]AA release in CHO cells with high expression and partial agonism when cAMP was evaluated. Hence, the compound can be used as a neutral antagonist only after careful assessment of its effect on the test system which is selected.

Constitutive activity of the native H_3R studied in vitro

The constitutive activity of the H_3 autoreceptor controlling [^{3}H]histamine release could be evidenced in cortical synaptosomes submitted to a strong depolarizing stimulus (40–55 mM K^+) in the mouse or rat. In agreement, both thioperamide and FUB 465 behaved as inverse agonists enhancing significantly the amine release, release being on the contrary reduced by the agonist imetit. Proxyfan, which alone did not affect [^{3}H]histamine release, blocked the opposite effects of either thioperamide and FUB 465 or imetit, therefore acting again as a neutral antagonist (Fig. 6). Clearly these responses could not involve endogenous histamine, and the endogenous amine level, even in the 55 mM K^+ medium, was two orders of magnitude less than its EC_{50} value as an agonist (5.3 ± 0.2 nM vs 200 ± 50 nM). That blockade of the H_3-autoreceptor stimulation by endogenous histamine does not significantly contribute to the releasing effect of drugs like thioperamide is also shown by i) the lack of

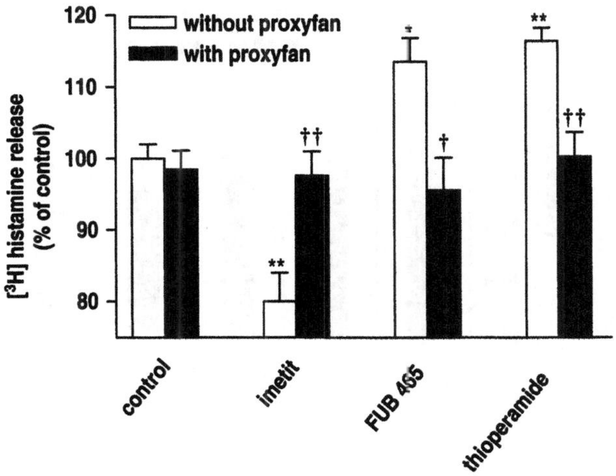

Fig. 6. Effects of H_3-receptor ligands on the K^+-induced release of [^{3}H]histamine from mouse cortical synaptosomes. Drugs (100 nM) were added with 55 mM K^+ and, when required, 10 μM proxyfan. Means ± SEM of 12–40 determinations from four separate experiments. *$P < 0.01$; **$P < 0.001$ vs control; †$P < 0.01$; ‡$P < 0.001$ vs without proxyfan (ANOVA followed by Newman-Keuls test) (reproduced with permission from Morisset et al., 2000)

releasing effect of proxyfan, acting here as a potent neutral antagonist, ii) the potent releasing effect of FUB 465, a potent inverse agonist at the H_3R mediating [^{3}H]AA release (EC_{50} ~ 10 nM) but weak neutral antagonist when opposed to histamine regarding the [^{3}H]amine release (K_i = 580 nM).

In addition, binding of the guanylnucleotide analogue [^{35}S]GTPγ[S] to mouse (or rat, not shown) cerebral membranes, demonstrated the coupling of the native H_3 receptor with G proteins (Clark and Hill, 1996), i.e. constitutive activity (Fig. 7). Thus, specific [^{35}S]GTPγ[S] binding was significantly reduced by FUB 465, ciproxifan or thioperamide, which were acting as inverse agonists as their effects were blocked by 1 μM proxyfan. Proxyfan also blocked the increase in binding elicited by imetit, but did not itself significantly affect binding, and was therefore acting again as a neutral antagonist in this test system. In contrast with this pattern, yohimbine, an inverse agonist at overexpressed or mutated α_2-adrenergic receptors, failed to decrease [^{35}S]GTPγ[S] binding to cerebral membranes, indicating that constitutive receptor activity is not an inevitable consequence of the experimental conditions required to evaluate the binding, as previously proposed (Costa et al., 1992).

The use of the [^{35}S]GTPγ[S] binding test allowed several other conclusions (Rouleau et al., 2002). Firstly, constitutive activity of the H_3R corresponds to the appearance of a high affinity binding site for the guanylnucleotide. Secondly, this constitutive activity of the H_3R was observed in all regions of the rat brain. Thirdly, the constitutive activity of the H_3R appears the highest among a large variety of other GPCRs (Fig. 8).

Among authors suggesting an inverse agonism at native GPCRs (De Ligt et al., 2000), Costa and Herz (1989) were pioneers by demonstrating for the

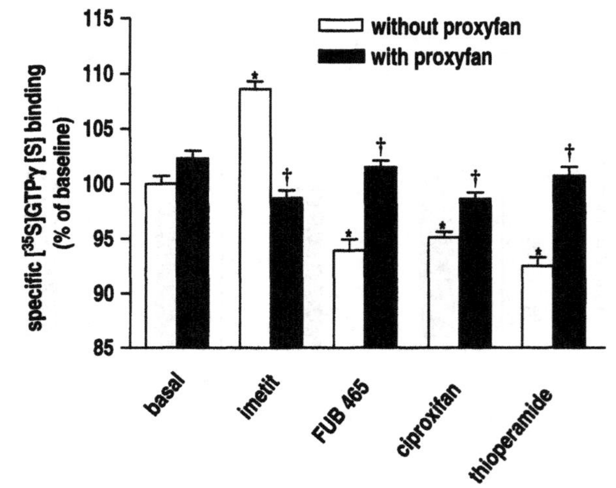

Fig. 7. Effects of H_3-receptor ligands (10 nM) on [^{35}S]GTPγ[S] binding to mouse cerebral cortical membranes in the presence or absence of 1 μM proxyfan. Means ± SEM of 9–24 determinations from four separate experiments. *P < 0.001 vs basal; †P < 0.01 vs without proxyfan (ANOVA followed by Newman-Keuls test) (reproduced with permission from Morisset et al., 2000)

first time that ICI-174864, an antagonist at the δ opioid receptor, behaved in fact as an inverse agonist at the δ opioid receptor endogenously expressed in NG 108-15 cells. However, the same authors reported that the inverse agonism induced by the drug occurred only in isolated membranes but not in intact cells (Costa et al., 1992). They suggested that constraints imposed by

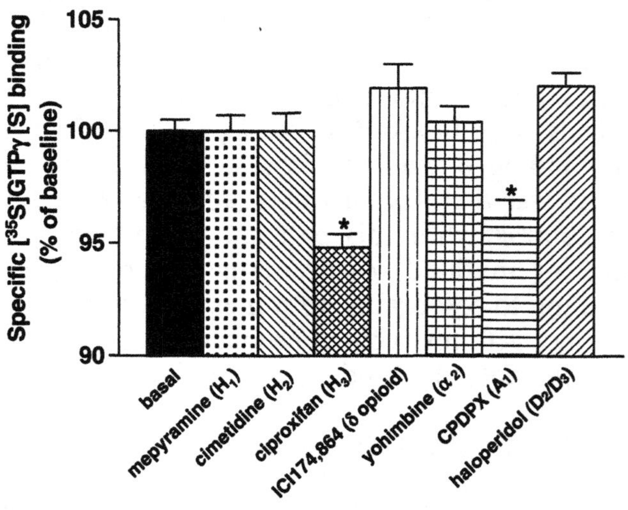

Fig. 8. Effects of inverse agonists at various G protein coupled-receptors on specific [^{35}S]GTPγ[S] binding to rat cerebral cortical membranes. Rat cerebral cortical membranes were incubated with 0.1 nM [^{35}S]]GTPγ[S] in the presence of the drugs at a 1 μM (mepyramine, cimetidine, ciproxifan, ICI-174,864 and CPDPX) or 0.1 μM (yohimbine and haloperidol) final concentration. Data represent means ± SEM of 8–39 determinations from two to four separate experiments. *P < 0.001 vs basal

cytosolic factors such as GTP prevent constitutive activity, making inevitable its observation in membranes upon separation from cytosol leading to removal of these factors. However, the present findings show that, in contrast to H_3R receptors, not all native receptors display constitutive activity in rat brain membranes. Indeed, in contrast to its inverse agonist effect on GTPase activity (Costa and Herz, 1989) and [^{35}S]GTPγ[S] binding (Szekeres and Traynor, 1997) in membranes of NG108-15 cells, ICI-174864 did not decrease [^{35}S]GTPγ[S] binding to membranes of rat cerebral cortex or striatum. These findings suggest that the threshold expression level for constitutive activity inherent to δ opioid receptors is not reached in the brain. The same interpretation may account for the apparent lack of effect of inverse agonists at D_2/D_3 dopamine, H_1 and H_2 histamine and α_2-adrenergic receptors, that we report here in brain membranes, in spite of the inverse agonism that they induce in cells (Nilsson and Eriksson, 1993; Griffon et al., 1996; Bakker et al., 2000; Alewijnse et al., 1998; Pauwels et al., 2000). It should be pointed out, however, that an apparent lack of inverse agonism does not furnish definitive evidence for the absence of constitutive activity since the intrinsic activity of a given inverse agonist is dependent on receptor systems and experimental conditions (Newman-Tancredi et al., 1997; Szekeres and Traynor, 1997; Pauwels et al., 1997, 2000; Audinot et al., 2001). Besides H_3Rs, A_1 adenosine receptors display a high constitutive activity in rat brain. Constitutive inhibition of adenylyl cyclase by A_1 adenosine receptors was previously shown using CPDPX. This drug known as a potent and highly selective antagonist, was acting as an inverse agonist not only at overexpressed receptors in CHO cells (Shryock et al., 1998) but also at endogenously expressed receptors of embryonic chick ventricular myocytes (Ma and Green, 1992). Although endogenous adenosine is present in high enough concentrations to stimulate [^{35}S]GTPγ[S] binding in rat brain sections (Laitinen and Jokinen, 1998), the decrease evoked by CPDPX in membranes is more likely to reflect high constitutive activity of cerebral A_1 receptors rather than antagonism of endogenous adenosine since it was observed after pretreatment of the membranes with adenosine deaminase.

In conclusion, the present study suggests that constitutive activity of native H_3Rs is one of the highest among GPCRs present in rat brain. Recombinant hH_3Rs also display high constitutive activity. The latter is easily detected at moderate concentrations, suggesting that it is present in human brain.

Constitutive activity of the native H_3R in brain in vivo

Three inverse agonists markedly enhanced cerebral histamine neuron activity in vivo, increasing by ~80% at maximum the levels of the histamine metabolite tele-methylhistamine (t-MeHA), a reliable marker of this activity (Fig. 9), and increasing histamine turnover as evaluated by the pargylin-induced t-MeHA accumulation in brain (not shown). This effect reflects an inverse agonist rather than the antagonist activity (towards endogenous histamine) of these ligands, as assumed so far (Arrang et al., 1987; Garbarg et al., 1989). In

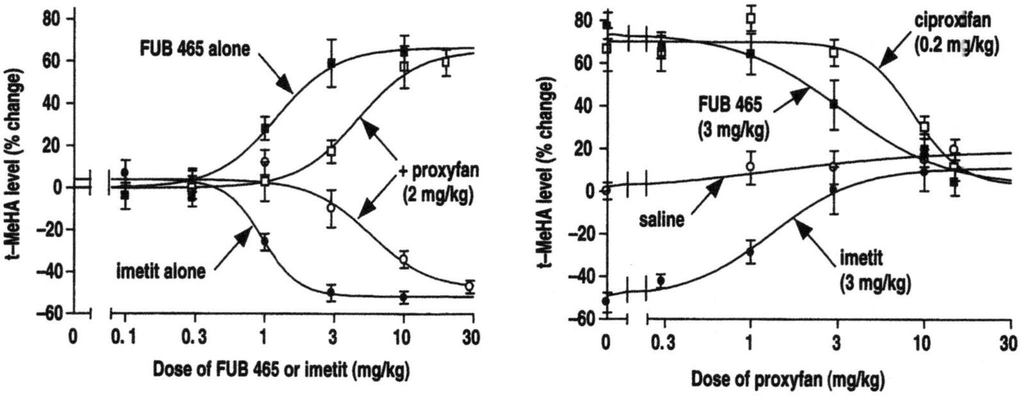

Fig. 9. Changes in brain t-MeHA levels in mice receiving H_3-receptor ligands (p.o.) and killed 90 min thereafter. Means ± SEM of 8–16 values expressed as percent change of values obtained in vehicle-treated mice (119 ± 4 ng/g) (reproduced with permission from Morisset et al., 2000)

agreement, the effect of FUB 465, obtained at a low dose (ED_{50} ~ 1 mg/kg, p.o.), was more consistent with its nanomolar potency as an inverse agonist than its micromolar potency as an antagonist. Moreover, the increases in t-MeHA level by FUB 465 and ciproxifan were competitively antagonized by proxyfan given at doses of ~2 mg/kg which also blocked the decrease in t-MeHA level induced by the agonist imetit. At these doses, proxyfan administered alone failed to affect significantly t-MeHA levels, indicating that it was acting as a neutral antagonist in vivo on a system regulated by H_3 receptors displaying constitutive activity. The small but significant increase (by ~20%) observed with proxyfan in doses above 10 mg/kg, might reflect its antagonist activity towards endogenous histamine.

Therapeutic implications

The best studied effect of H_3R inverse agonists is to enhance histamine neuron activity and histamine release in brain, a result of their interaction at the autoreceptor, although the majority of H_3Rs in brain are, in fact, heteroreceptors.

Hence the question to be raised is that of clinical implication of brain histamine neurons in psychiatric diseases.

Overdose of a variety of classical H_1-antagonists was repeatedly reported to result in toxic psychoses with hallucinations resembling schizophrenia and the hallucinogenic potential of these drugs has even led to abuse (Sangalli, 1997).

On the other hand, metamphetamine, a drug with hallucinogenic potential and to which schizophrenic patients seem hyper-responsive, releases histamine in rodent brain areas, an indirect effect mediated by stimulation of D_2 and not D_3 dopamine receptors (Ito et al., 1996; Morisset et al., 1999). Even more, endogenous dopamine appears to exert a tonic stimulation of histamine neurons since typical neuroleptics, e.g. haloperidol, decrease their activity. In contrast, atypical neuroleptics, e.g. clozapine, enhance histamine turnover, an effect related to 5-HT_2 receptor blockade and possibly underlying their procognitive properties (Morisset et al., 1999). The locomotor activation elicited in rodents by amphetamine and other dopaminergic agonists is attenuated by H_3-receptor blockade (Clapham and Kilpatrick, 1994). Repeated amphetamine administration in rodents which results in behavioral sensitization to dopamine agonists, a cardinal feature of schizophrenia, is accompanied by enhanced histamine release which presumably reflects an enhanced tonic dopaminergic influence on histaminergic neurons (Ito et al., 1996; Morisset et al., 1999). Interestingly, in one comprehensive study, an enhanced level of t-methylhistamine, the major histamine metabolite, was detected in the CSF of schizophrenic patients, either treated or non treated by neuroleptics (Prell et al., 1995).

In several open studies famotidine, an H_2-antagonist, was found to improve schizophrenic patients, a finding which remains to be confirmed in control studies. A previous claim of association between polymorphisms of the H_2-receptor gene and schizophrenia could not be confirmed (Ito et al., 2000).

These various observations, although not easily forming a coherent picture, suggest that inverse agonists at the H_3R might be useful in schizophrenia treatment.

Neuropathological studies have documented a deficit in histaminergic neurotransmission in Alzheimer's disease (AD). In some, but not all, cortical areas (e.g. frontal or temporal cortex) of AD brains, there is a decrease of histamine and histidine decarboxylase levels that may reach up to ~50% (Panula et al., 1998) and the expression of the hdc gene in neurons of the tuberomammillary nucleus is also reduced (S. Trottier, personal communication). Decreased histaminergic input may affect cholinergic neuron activity in nucleus basilis (Khateb et al., 1995) and acetylcholine release in cortical areas.

Taking into account an additional direct positive influence of histamine on attention and memory, this indicates that enhancing histaminergic neurotransmission may constitute a novel symptomatic therapeutic approach to AD. Interestingly the drug tacrine was even more potent in inhibiting histamine-N-methyltransferase, the main histamine-metabolizing enzyme, than acetylcholinesterase (Morisset et al., 1996).

All above observations suggest that inverse agonists of the H_3R represent a class of novel candidates with potential in psychiatric and other diseases.

References

Alewijnse AE, Smit MJ, Hoffmann M, Verzijl D, Timmerman H, Leurs R (1998) Constitutive activity and structural instability of the wild-type human H_2 receptor. J Neurochem 71: 799–807

Arrang JM, Garbarg M, Schwartz JC (1983) Auto-inhibition of brain histamine release mediated by a novel class (H_3) of histamine receptor. Nature 302: 832–837

Arrang JM, Garbarg M, Lancelot JC, Lecomte JM, Pollard H, Robba M, Schunack W, Schwartz JC (1987) Highly potent and selective ligands for histamine H_3-receptors. Nature 327: 117–123

Audinot V, Newman-Tancredi A, Millan MJ (2001) Constitutive activity at serotonin 5-HT_{1D} receptors: detection by homologous GTPgS versus [^{35}S]-GTPgS binding isotherms. Neuropharmacol 40: 57–64

Bakker RA, Wieland K, Timmerman H, Leurs R (2000) Constitutive activity of the histamine H_1 receptor reveals inverse agonism of histamine H_1 receptor antagonists. Eur J Pharmacol 387: R5–R7

Chen G, Way J, Armour S, Watson C, Queen K, Jayawickreme CK, Chen WJ, Kenakin T (2000) Use of constitutive G protein-coupled receptor activity for drug discovery. Mol Pharmacol 57: 125–134

Chidiac P, Hebert TE, Valiquette M, Dennis M, Bouvier M (1994) Inverse agonism activity of β-adrenergic antagonists. Mol Pharmacol 45: 490–499

Claeysen S, Sebben M, Becamel C, Bockaert J, Dumuis A (1999) Novel brain-specific 5-HT_4 receptor splice variants show marked constitutive activity: role of the C-terminal intracellular domain. Mol Pharmacol 55: 910–920

Clapham J, Kilpatrick GJ (1994) Thioperamide, the selective histamine H_3 receptor antagonist, attenuates stimulant-induced locomotor activity in the mouse. Eur J Pharmacol 259: 107–114

Clark EA, Hill SJ (1995) Differential effect of sodium ions and guanine nucleotides on the binding of thioperamide and clobenpropit to histamine H_3-receptors in rat cerebral cortical membranes. Br J Pharmacol 114: 357–362

Clark EA, Hill SJ (1996) Sensitivity of histamine H_3 receptor agonist-stimulated [^{35}S]GTP gamma[S] binding to pertussis toxin. Eur J Pharmacol 296: 223–225

Costa T, Herz A (1989) Antagonists with negative intrinsic activity at delta opioid receptors coupled to GTP-binding proteins. Proc Natl Acad Sci USA 86: 7321–7325

Costa T, Ogino Y, Munson PJ, Onaran O, Rodbard D (1992) Drug efficacy at guanine nucleotide-binding regulatory protein-linked receptors: thermodynamic interpretation of negative antagonism and of receptor activity in the absence of ligand. Mol Pharmacol 41: 549–560

de Ligt RAF, Kourounakis AP, Ijzerman AP (2000) Inverse agonism at G protein-coupled receptors: (patho)physiological relevance and implications for drug discovery. Br J Pharmacol 130: 1–12

Garbarg M, Trung Tuong MD, Gros C, Schwartz JC (1989) Effects of histamine H_3-receptor ligands on various biochemical indices of histaminergic neuron activity in rat brain. Eur J Pharmacol 164: 1–11

Griffon N, Pilon C, Sautel F, Schwartz JC, Sokoloff P (1996) Antipsychotics with inverse agonist activity at the dopamine D_3 receptor. J Neural Transm 103: 1163–1175

Ito C, Onodera K, Sakurai E, Sato M, Watanabe T (1996) Effects of dopamine antagonists on neuronal histamine release in the striatum of rats subjected to acute and chronic treatments with methamphetamine. J Pharmacol Exp Ther 279: 271–276

Ito C, Morisset S, Krebs MO, Olié JP, Lôo H, Poirier MF, Lannfelt L, Schwartz JC, Arrang JM (2000) Histamine H_2 receptor gene variants: lack of association with schizophrenia. Mol Psychiat 5: 159–164

Kenakin TP (1997) Pharmacological analysis of drug receptor interaction. Lippincott-Raven, New York

Khateb A, Fort P, Pegna A, Jones BE, Muhlethaler M (1995) Cholinergic nucleus basilis neurons are excited by histamine in vitro. Neuroscience 69: 495–506

Laitinen JT, Jokinen M (1998) Guanosine 5′-(γ-[^{35}S]thio)triphosphate autoradiography allows selective detection of histamine H_3 receptor-dependent G protein activation in rat brain tissue sections. J Neurochem 71: 808–816

Lefkowitz RJ, Cotecchia S, Samama P, Costa T (1993) Constitutive activity of receptors coupled to guanine nucleotide regulatory proteins. Trends Pharmacol Sci 14: 303–307

Leurs R, Smit MJ, Alewijnse AE, Timmerman H (1998) Agonist-independent regulation of constitutively active G-protein-coupled receptors. Trends Biochem Sci 23: 418–422

Ligneau X, Garbarg M, Vizuete ML, Diaz J, Purand K, Stark H, Schunack W, Schwartz JC (1994) [^{125}I]Iodoproxyfan, a new antagonist to label and visualize cerebral histamine H_3 receptors. J Pharmacol Exp Ther 271: 452–459

Ligneau X, Lin JS, Vanni-Mercier G, Jouvet M, Muir JL, Ganellin CR, Stark H, Elz S, Schunack W, Schwartz JC (1998) Neurochemical and behavioral effects of ciproxifan, a potent histamine H_3-receptor antagonist. J Pharmacol Exp Ther 287: 658–666

Lovenberg TW, Roland BL, Wilson SJ, Jiang X, Pyati J, Huvar A, Jackson MR, Erlander MG (1999) Cloning and functional expression of the human histamine H_3 receptor. Mol Pharmacol 55: 1101–1107

Ma H, Green RD (1992) Modulation of cardiac cyclic AMP metabolism by adenosine receptor agonists and antagonists. Mol Pharmacol 42: 831–837

Milligan G, Bond R (1997) Inverse agonism and the regulation of receptor number. Trends Pharmacol Sci 18: 468–474

Milligan G, Bond R, Lee M (1995) Inverse agonism: pharmacological curiosity or potential therapeutic strategy? Trends Pharmacol Sci 16: 10–13

Morisset S, Traiffort E, Schwartz JC (1996) Inhibition of histamine versus acetylcholine metabolism as a mechanism of tacrine activity. Eur J Pharmacol 315: R1–R2

Morisset S, Sahm UG, Traiffort E, Tardivel-Lacombe J, Arrang JM, Schwartz JC (1999) Atypical neuroleptics enhance histamine turnover in brain via 5-hydroxytryptamine$_{2A}$ receptor blockade. J Pharmacol Exp Ther 288: 590–596

Morisset S, Rouleau A, Ligneau X, Gbahou F, Tardivel-Lacombe J, Stark H, Schunack W, Ganellin CR, Schwartz JC, Arrang JM (2000) High constitutive activity of native H_3 receptors regulates histamine neurons in brain. Nature 408: 860–864

Newman-Tancredi A, Conte C, Chaput C, Verriele L, Millan MJ (1997) Agonist and inverse agonist efficacy at human recombinant serotonin 5-HT_{1A} receptors as a function of receptor: G-protein stoichiometry. Neuropharmacol 36: 451–459

Newman-Tancredi A, Audinot V, Moreira C, Verriele L, Millan MJ (2000) Inverse agonism and constitutive activity as functional correlates of serotonin h5-HT_{1B} receptor/G-protein stoichiometry. Mol Pharmacol 58: 1042–1049

Nilsson CL, Eriksson E (1993) Haloperidol increases prolactin release and cyclic AMP formation in vitro: inverse agonism at dopamine D_2 receptors? J Neural Transm 92: 213–220

Panula P, Rinne J, Kuokkanen K, Eriksson KS, Sallmen T, Kalimo H, Relja M (1998) Neuronal histamine deficit in Alzheimer's disease. Neuroscience 82: 993–997

Pauwels PJ, Tardif S, Wurch T, Colpaert FC (1997) Stimulated [^{35}S]-GTPγS binding by 5-HT_{1A} receptor agonists in recombinant cell lines: modulation of apparent efficacy by G-protein activation state. Naunyn Schmiedebergs Arch Pharmacol 356: 551–561

Pauwels PJ, Tardif S, Wurch T, Colpaert FC (2000) Facilitation of constitutuve α_{2A}-adrenoceptor activity by both single amino acid mutation (thr^{373}lys) and $G_{\alpha o}$ protein coexpression: evidence for inverse agonism. J Pharmacol Exp Ther 292: 654–663

Pozvek G, Hilton JM, Quiza M, Houssami S, Sexton PM (1997) Structure/function relationships of calcitonin analogues as agonists, antagonists, or inverse agonists in a constitutively activated receptor cell system. Mol Pharmacol 51: 658–665

Prell GD, Green JP, Kaufmann CA, Khandelwal JK, Morrishow AM, Kirch DG, Linnoila M, Wyatt RJ (1995) Histamine metabolites in cerebrospinal fluid of patients with chronic schizophrenia: their relationship to levels of other aminergic transmitters and ratings of symptoms. Schizophr Res 14: 93–104

Rouleau A, Ligneau X, Tardivel-Lacombe J, Morisset S, Gbahou F, Schwartz JC, Arrang JM (2002) Histamine H_3-receptor-mediated [^{35}S]GTPγ[S] binding: evidence for constitutive activity of the recombinant and native rat and human H_3 receptors. Br J Pharmacol 135: 383–392

Samama P, Cotecchia S, Costa T, Lefkowitz RJ (1993) A mutation-induced activated state of the β_2-adrenergic receptor. Extending the ternary complex model. J Biol Chem 268: 4625–4636

Sangalli BC (1997) Role of the central histaminergic neuronal system in the CNS toxicity of the first generation H_1-antagonists. Prog Neurobiol 52: 145–157

Shryock JC, Ozeck MJ, Belardinelli L (1998) Inverse agonists and neutral antagonists of recombinant human A_1 adenosine receptors stably expressed in chinese hamster ovary cells. Mol Pharmacol 53: 886–893

Strange P (2002) Mechanisms of inverse agonism at G-protein-coupled receptors. Trends Pharmacol Sci 23: 89–95

Szekeres PG, Traynor JR (1997) Delta opioid modulation of the binding of guanosine-5′-O-(3-[^{35}S]thio)triphosphate to NG108-15 cell membranes: characterization of agonist and inverse agonist effects. J Pharmacol Exp Ther 283: 1276–1284

Tardivel-Lacombe J, Rouleau A, Héron A, Morisset S, Pillot C, Cochois V, Schwartz JC, Arrang JM (2000) Cloning and cerebral expression of the guinea pig histamine H_3 receptor: evidence for two isoforms. NeuroReport 11: 755–759

Authors' address: J.-C. Schwartz, Unité de Neurobiologie et Pharmacologie Moléculaire (U.573) INSERM, Centre Paul Broca, 2ter rue d'Alésia, F-75014 Paris, France, e-mail: schwartz@broca.inserm.fr

J Neural Transm (2003) [Suppl] 64: 17–34

The role of peptides in treatment of psychiatric disorders

F. Holsboer

Max Planck Institute of Psychiatry, Munich, Federal Republic of Germany

Summary. About 25 years ago the observation that neuropeptides serve as signalling molecules in the nervous system generated great expectations for drug industry. In this article the progress made since then in exploiting neuropeptide systems pharmacologically in psychiatry is highlighted.

In affective disorders a number of neuropeptides seem to be causally involved in development and course of illness, especially corticotropin releasing hormone (CRH), vasopressin (AVP) and substance P, whose receptors are now targeted with small molecules designed to reduce depressive and anxiety symptoms. Although not exactly neuropeptides, also neurotrophins, may have a distinct role in antidepressant action and possibly also in causation of depression. Schizophrenia-like symptoms are caused by neurotensin (NT), supporting the notion that drugs interfering with NT systems are potential antipsychotics. Finally, sleep disorders, currently treated with hypnotics, that have serious adverse effects can be targeted with neuropeptides. According to the work by Axel Steiger several neuropeptides even if peripherally administered produce improvements of quality of sleep.

All these observations call for intensified application of novel research tools necessary to exploit the potential of neuropeptide systems as psychopharmaceutical targets.

Introduction

The neuropeptide hypothesis was originally championed by Dorothy Krieger (1983) and David de Wied (1993), but the tools available 10–20 years ago where inappropriate to prove the concept and to fully exploit neuropeptide systems pharmacologically. In this treatise I will not exhaustively refer to all neuropeptides considered to be involved in psychiatric syndromes. Instead a number of examples is given illustrating the promises and caveats of neuropeptide-related pharmacology.

Peptides are small proteins and if produced in neurons they are called neuropeptides, which serve neurotransmitter-like function in the nervous system. Some neuropeptides are directly released into the blood by neurons and act systemically as hormones. Many neuropeptides are coexpressed and cosecreted in classic neurotransmitter neurons, such as norepinephrine neurons. A particularly important difference between classic neurotransmitter signalling and neuropeptide signalling is that only the latter can convey a signal over long distances. When a classic neurotransmitter is released into the synaptic cleft, most of this small molecule is rapidly taken up and returned to the presynaptic terminal via a cell membrane located transporter (e.g. serotonin reuptake transporter). Neuropeptides, in contrast, are not rapidly cleared from the synapse and their action is terminated by peptidases that reside in extracellular membranes. Because of this long distance signalling property and anatomic locations of many neuropeptides do not correspond precisely to the locations of their receptors. This neuroanatomical mismatch has created considerable confusion. Also the lack of pharmacological tools, e.g. peptide agonists and antagonists that cross the blood-brain barrier has hampered the field as much as the difficulty to quantitate release of neuropeptides in specific brain areas. The current availability of mouse mutants where certain neuropeptides are over- or underexpressed or where the corresponding receptors are genetically deleted has been a major advance for the field. This and new developments in dynamic combinatorial chemistry directly addressing the respective target and self-screening the available libraries promises a flurry of potentially valuable new leads from which hopefully new drugs well emerge.

Targeting the stress-hormone system to treat affective disorders — a case for CRH and vasopressin

Elevated activity of the hypothalamic-pituitary-adrenocortical (HPA) system in affective disorders has long been a mainstay in the search for causality and treatment of depression and anxiety. Originally it was thought that excessive production and release of cortisol, which enters easily the brain may account for some of the signs and symptoms of depression. This view stemmed from classic work by Manfred Bleuler in Zürich, carefully characterizing patients with endocrine diseases such as Cushing's syndrome or patients treated with corticosteroids for other reasons, e.g. inflammations. Not before studies monitoring HPA-status in depressed patients longitudinally it became clear that central nervous system controlled stress responses have a dual action: While CRH released from neurons in the hypothalamus may produce hypercortisolism via the HPA-system, CRH released from other brain loci and binding at the prefrontal cortex, amygdala, hippocampus, locus coeruleus etc. can produce stress-adaptive responses that when these continue over time they result in depression or anxiety disorders. The key argument for this hypothesis came from studies initiated in the 80ties measuring CRH in the cerebrospinal fluid (CSF) and CRH-binding sites in the prefrontal cortex and from neuroendocrine studies in depressives which, in essence, supported the notion that CRH is elevated in depression (review: Holsboer, 1999). To challenge the question whether CRH has other effects than eliciting stress hormones, numerous studies admininistered CRH centrally and showed that CRH precipitates a number of behavioral changes comparable to an anxiogenic stressor (see Fig. 1). Studies using antisense probes suppressing

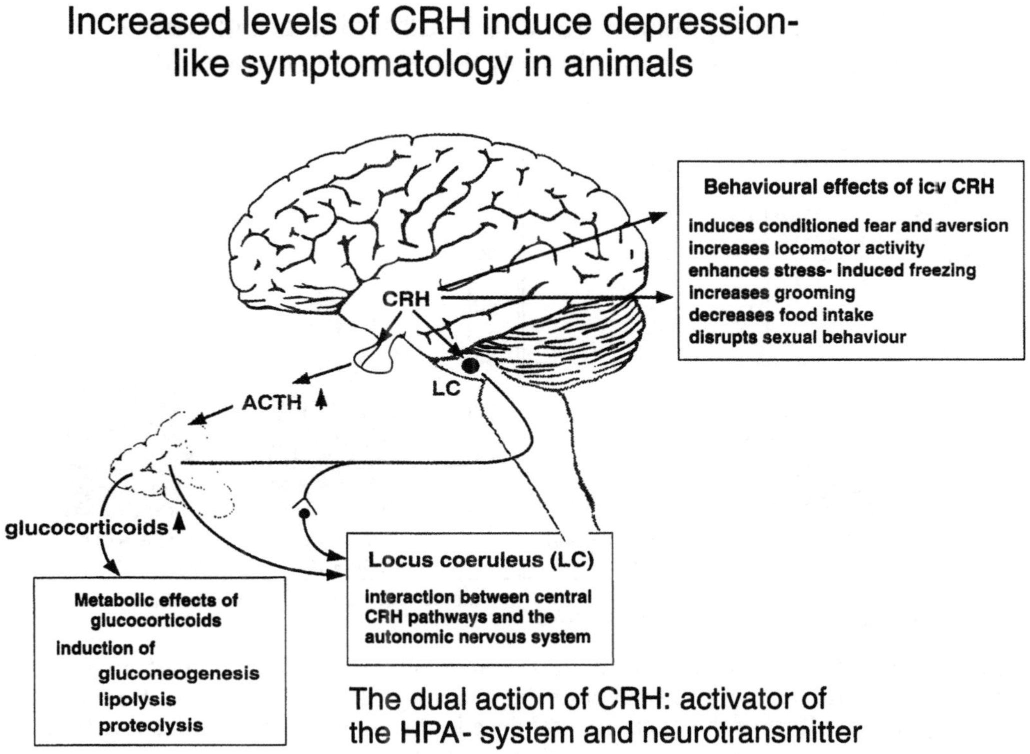

Fig. 1. Summarization of preclinical and clinical evidence supporting the hypothesis that CRH is a key neuropeptide accounting for many signs and symptoms characteristic for stress-related diseases, such as depression and anxiety

CRHmRNA conversion into CRH as well as studies using mice that overexpress CRH all corroborated a causal pathogenetic role of CRH in depression and anxiety (review: Landgraf, 2001).

Two CRH receptor subtypes CRHR1 and CRHR2 with distinct anatomical localization and receptor pharmacology have been identified. The CRHR1 is a protein containing 415 amino acids and comprises 7 putative transmembrane spanning regions similar to that of other G-protein coupled receptors (GPCR). The CRHR2-receptor encodes a 411-amino acid GPCR with about 70% homology to the CRHR1. The CRHR2 exists in two different splice variants, CRHR2A (predominantly expressed in the brain) and CRHR2B (predominantly expressed in the periphery). CRH is relatively selective for CRHR1 over CRHR2 but another neuropeptide, urocortin (UCN) is bound to both receptors with high affinity (review: Reul and Holsboer, 2002). Recently two novel selective ligands were discovered, stresscopin-related peptide, UCNII and stresscopin UCNIII) that selectively bind to CRHR2 (Hsu and Hsueh, 2001). The function of these two neuropeptides in relation to behavior needs studies with animal models where expression of stresscopin and its related receptor are genetically modified. The ultimate decision which receptor should be targeted to prevent pathological behavioral responses secondary to continued overexpression of CRH was provided from studies

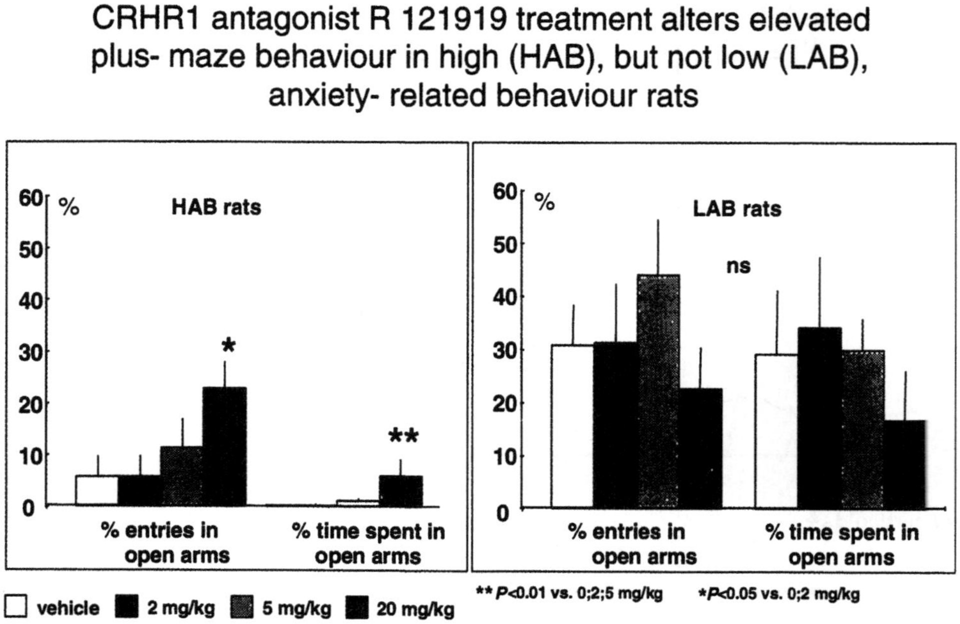

Fig. 2. Treatment of rats with high innate anxiety show a reduction of anxiety-like behavior when treated with a nonpeptide, high affinity CRHR1 antagonist. Note that the dose-dependent effect of the experimental drug is absent among rats selectively bred for low anxiety-like behavior (Keck et al., 2002)

using a mouse mutant where the CRHR1 was deleted. These mice were less anxious when stressed (Timpl et al., 1998) and showed other behavioral symptoms characteristic for defective response to stress. For example, when exposed to enduring stress these animals consumed much more ethanol than controls (Sillaber et al., 2002).

The group by Rainer Landgraf generated a rat strain with increased and decreased innate anxiety through selective breeding (Liebsch et al., 1998). Keck et al. (2001a) treated these high anxiety (HAB) and low anxiety (LAB) rats with R121919 (formerly NBI 30775) a selective water soluble CRHR1 antagonist which binds with high affinity ($K_i \sim 3$ nM) to cloned human CRHR1. Only HAB but not LAB rats responded with a dose dependent reduction of anxiety-like behavior (see Fig. 2) which is in agreement with Tomas Hökfelts (1991) hypothesis that neuropeptides are only secreted if the neuronal firing rate has exceeded a certain level (see Fig. 3). Encouraged by these data a first open-label study in 20 patients with major depression was conducted. The doses used in the study (5–40 mg/day or 40–80 mg/day for 30 days) were well tolerated and had prompted no adverse effects. Interestingly, these dosages did not affect ACTH or cortisol levels at baseline or following a CRH challenge test (Zobel et al., 2000). This agrees with autoradiographic studies by Keck et al. (2001a) who showed that even at high antagonist dosages replacing CRH throughout the brain still leaves sufficient amounts of functional CRHR1 at the pituitary. In this clinical study both, anxiety and depression scores, dropped significantly (Zobel, 2000). In fact, these

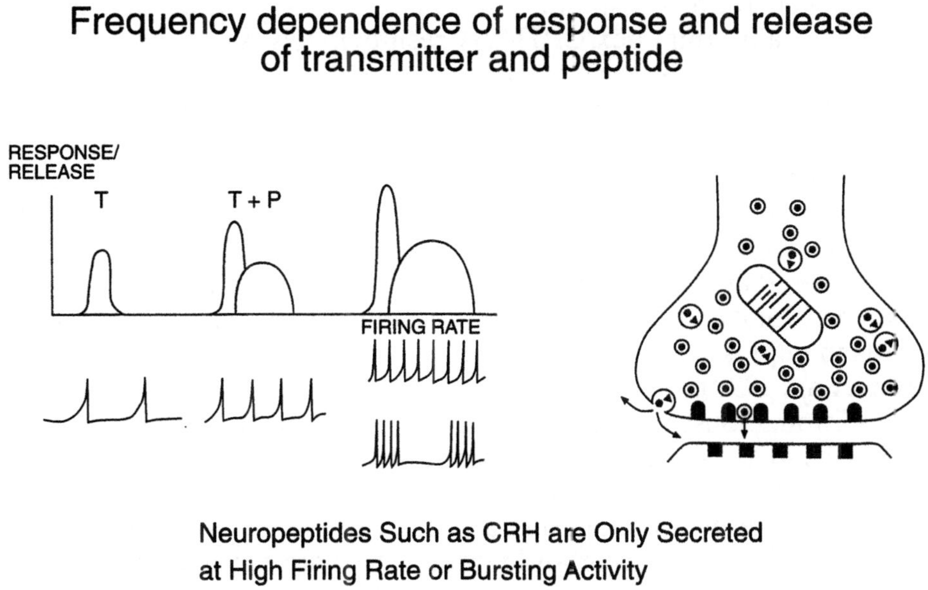

Fig. 3. Thomas Hökfelt's hypothesis that neuropeptides are hypersecreted under conditions of increased neuronal firing which prevails under pathophysiological conditions has recently been supported by preclinical (Keck et al., 2002) and clinical studies (Zobel et al., 2000) using a nonpeptide small-molecule that antagonising the effects of CRH hypersecretion of CRH1-receptors

changes were comparable with historical data from a controlled study using paroxetine. While this particular product (R121919) is no longer pursued several pharmaceutical companies now emphasize drug discovery and drug development projects aiming at CRHR1 antagonists.

The rats with high innate anxiety (HAB rats) hypersecrete vasopressin. Vasopressin itself is not only involved in cognition but also in emotionality and suppressing V_{1A}-receptor via antisense targeting reduced both, cognitive function and anxiety-like behavior (Landgraf et al., 1995). While the finding by Reul et al. (1993, 1994) has corroborated that antidepressants increase mineralo- and glucocorticosteroid receptor function (review: Holsboer and Barden, 1996), a more recent study by Keck et al. (unpublished) provided a surprising result. These authors showed that paroxetine and SSRI when given to high-anxiety (HAB) rats decreases vasopressin production in the hypothalamus. A potential role of vasopressin/V_{1A}-receptor signalling in affective disorders is also suggested by a study of Keck et al. (2001b) using the dexamethasone/CRH-test. This neuroendocrine test administers a low oral dexamethasone dose (1.5 mg, 23.00 h) followed by a CRH challenge (100 µg, 15.00 h). Only patients with depression, either during an episode or with impeding risk for relapse show excessive release of ACTH and cortisol in the context of the test (review: Holsboer, 2000). Only HAB but not LAB rats show the same hormonal response pattern as patients with depression. Both, HAB rats and depressed patients when treated with antidepressants show a gradual normalization of the dex/CRH-test result. Early studies by von Bardeleben et al.

(1985) and von Bardeleben and Holsboer (1989) submitted that the pathophysiology of abnormal dex/CRH-test results involves vasopressin hypersecretion. This hypothesis was later corroborated by Dinan et al. (1999) and by Dick Swaab's group showing increased coexpression of CRH and vasopressin in the hypothalami of depressed humans (Purba et al., 1996; Raadsheer et al., 1994). From a study by Keck et al. (unpublished) it can be concluded that paroxetine reduces vasopressin in the hypothalamus. However, it is unclear whether this antidepressant-induced reduction of vasopressin is causally related to reduced anxiety-like behavior in rats or reduced depression scores in depressives. Notably, CRH concentrations in the CSF are reduced by antidepressants in depressives, while the CSF vasopressin levels remain unchanged (Heuser et al., 1998).

In addition, mouse mutants with deletions of CRHR1 or of both CRHR1 and CRHR2, hypersecrete vasopressin, but nevertheless show decreased or unchanged anxiety-like behavior (Müller et al., 2001; Preil et al., 2001). Thus it is clear that the neuroendocrine aspect of excessive HPA-activity and its gradual normalization during antidepressant treatment involves initially increased vasopressin secretion from the hypothalamus which is reduced during drug treatment. Whether a similar reduction of vasopressin in other brain areas accounts for resolution of depressive psychopathology remains unclear. Nevertheless, the behavioral data triggered the development of nonpeptide vasopressin antagonists directed against V_{1A} and V_{1B} receptors, both of which have neuroanatomical locations (amygdala, septum, hippocampus, hypothalamus) making then interesting drug targets. Recently a study by Griebel et al. (2002) using a pyrrolidine carboxamide which selectively antagonises V_{1B}-receptors was administered to rats and mice. Administering the elevated plus maze-test in rats and the dark/light-test in mice, the forced swim test in rats and chronic mild stress test, all well established tests to discover possible antidepressive or anxiolytic effects, the new V_{1B}-receptor antagonist displayed a behavioral profile consistent with an anxiolytic or antidepressant like action under clinical conditions in humans. Notably the animal tests used conformed the standards under which currently available antidepressants were previously identified through screening tests. Future results from clinical development programs will show whether innovative pharmacological leads can be detected when using test models designed for previous (and overcome) drugs. Note that CRHR1-antagonists worked only among HAB rats having an innate (i.e. genetically imprinted) psychopathology. Moreover, focussing only upon V_{1B}-receptors might be premature as both, neuroanatomical distribution at V_{1A}-receptors and behavioral studies, by Landgraf et al. (1995) favour the search for clinically feasible V_{1A} receptor antagonists.

Substance P and NK1 receptor antagonists

Substance P belongs to the family of tachykinins and among these family members it is by far the most concentrated in the human brain. Its preferred receptor in the brain is the NK1-receptor which has a widespread neu-

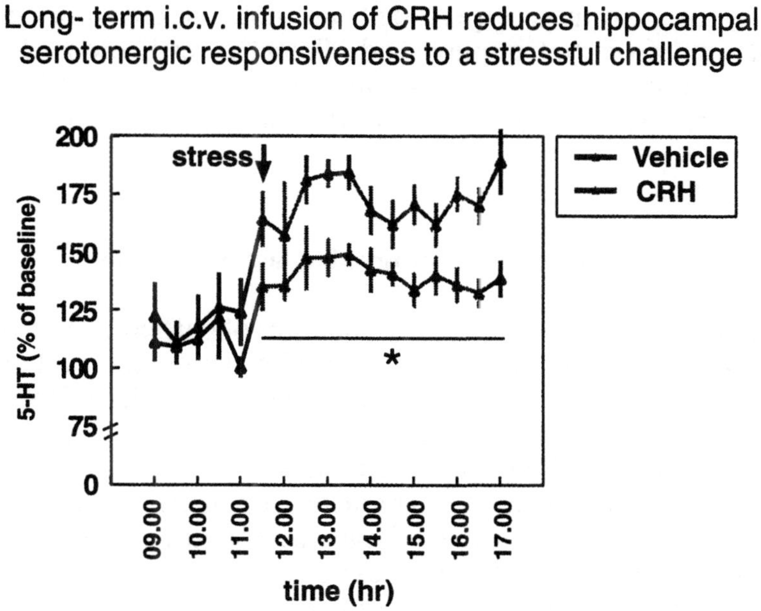

Fig. 4. An experiment by Astrid Linthorst (1995) illustrates that neuropeptidergic and aminergic systems are intrinsically intertwined. Long-term exposure to CRH can blunt stress elicited hippocampal serotonin release

roanatomical distribution including many loci in the limbic system (e.g. amygdala, septum, hypothalamus) and the brain stem (locus coeruleus, raphe nuclei). The former locations suggest a role for substance P/NK1-signalling for emotionality, the latter location for monoamine interactions (Chawla et al., 1997). A study by Teixera et al. (1996) suggested that central administration of substance P produces anxiety-like behavior while administration of an NK1-receptor antagonist proved to be anxiolytic in rats (File, 2000). The latter finding is in accord with a study by Santarelli (2001) showing that genetic and pharmacological disruption of the NK1-receptor gene results in decreased anxiety-like behavior. This study also highlighted how intrinsically intertwined monoaminergic and neuropeptidergic transmitter systems might be as they showed that NK1-receptor disruption increases serotonergic function. Along the same line Astrid Linthorst's group (Penalva et al., 2002) reported that in case of reduced CRHR1-receptor function, i.e. in heterozygous and homozygous CRHR1 null mutants the stress induced hippocampal 5-HT surge is increased (see Fig. 4). Translated into drug therapy this means that NK1- or CRHR1-receptor antagonists may increase serotonergic neurotransmission. A recent clinical trial by Kramer et al. (1998) included 213 patients that were randomly assigned to an NK1-receptor antagonist (NK 869) paroxetine (an SSRI, 20 mg) or placebo. In fact, paroxetine and NK 869 were equally effective and superior to placebo. This report prompted reevaluation of basic studies employing a variety of tests including ultrasound vocalizations of neonatal mice separated from their mothers which were decreased in mutants with disrupted NK1-receptors. Similar effects were also observed among guinea pigs when treated with standard antidepressants. While not immediately intuitive these experiments are now backed up by more established tests and from yet unpublished clinical investigations. In all, there seems to be a convergence of results that support the view that NK1-receptor antagonists are experimental drugs worthwhile to be studied in affective disorders.

Brain derived neurotrophic factor (BDNF)

BDNF is a peptide synthesized in the cell bodies of particular neurons and glia most abundantly in the hippocampus, where its expression level exceeds that of nerve growth factor 50 fold. In contrast to neuropeptides BDNF (as well as other neurotrophic factors) produces its effects by activation of tyrosine kinases which may be either intrinsic to their receptors (Trk-receptors) or separate proteins. One of the best characterized neurotrophin-activated signal transduction pathways is the *m*itogen-*a*ctivated *p*rotein (MAP) kinase cascade which includes ERK (an *e*xtracellular signal-*r*egulated protein *k*inase) as a key step (Chang and Karin, 2001). The activity of ERK/MAP kinase was reported to be decreased in the brain of suicide victims (Dwivedi et al., 2001). Similarly, hippocampal BDNF expression is suppressed in stressed rats (Smith et al., 1995) while expression of the BDNF receptor TrkB is enhanced (Nibuya at al., 1999). These findings have been linked with brain-imaging studies which demonstrated reduced hippocampal volumes in depression (Sheline et al., 1996, 1999; Bremner et al., 2000). While these interesting neuroradiological observations not necessarily reflect decreased hippocampal BDNF, some molecular pharmacological findings are of note as antidepressants where found to increase BDNF concentrations in the dentate gyrus, hilus and supragranular regions of the hippocampus (Chen et al., 2001). These effects were also seen in rats and are supposed to be mediated through phosphorylated *c*yclo-AMP *r*esponse *e*lement *b*inding protein (CREB) which transactivates BDNF gene expression (Thome et al., 2000) through binding to a CRE (*c*yclo-AMP *r*esponse *e*lement) in the BDNF gene promoter. Such a response element is also part of the CRH gene promoter (Spengler et al., 1992), pointing to a commonality of nuclear mechanisms once relevant kinases (protein kinase A, ERK) are activated through postreceptor signalling cascades. The observed suppression of BDNF following stress and its increase following antidepressant treatment including electroconvulsive shocks in rats has challenged the question whether BDNF itself may convey the mood elevating effect of antidepressants. While it seems clear that antidepressants promote CREB phosphorylation (at Serine, 133) a recent study by Ronald Dumans group used two established animal models of depression: Shirayama et al. (2002) used the learned helplessness (LH) rat model and the forced swim test (FST) and infused BDNF into the dentate gyrus of these animals. This area was chosen because there BDNF concentration changes in response to stress and drugs at a most profound degree. After dosages between 0.25 μg–1.0 μg in both tests long-term and persistent antidepressant-like effects were seen in both paradigms, the LH and the FST, supporting the notion that BDNF increase accounts for the behavioral effects observed after antidepressants. Heterocygous mice with BDNF gene knock out, however, did not exhibit any behavioral abnormality, although their hippocampal BDNF content is reduced (Montkowski et al., 1997) and although they have reduced long term potentiation in the CA1 area of the hippocampus (Korte et al., 1995; Kovalchuk et al., 2002). The latter phenomenon is thought to be a correlate of hippocampus mediated cognitive capacity. Another twist in the CREB/BDNF hypothesis is a study by Conti et al. (2002) who replicated the behavioral effect of antidepressants upon the FST in CREB-deficient mice which responded similar as wild-type mice. In these animals the behavioral effect of antidepressant was not associated with increased BDNF, confirming CREB as an upstream regulator of BDNF. Both molecules, CREB and BDNF, are apparently not necessary to produce antidepressant-elicited behavioral changes. Nevertheless, if CREB is present, it is possible that antidepressant-induced phosphorylation results in increased BDNF synthesis. In this context the most provocative aspect is whether antidepressants contribute to adult neurogenesis and whether this effect is contributing to their clinical action. While it is outside the scope of this treatise it is of note that neurogenesis in the adult hippocampus is restricted to the subgranular zone and newborn neurons appear to migrate only as far as the nearby dentate granule layer. In as much this neurogenesis accounts for psychotropic action of antidepressants is still an open question. Even more interesting seems to me to unravel by which kind of mechanism social stress might suppress adult granule cell proliferation and retraction of apical dendrites of CA3 pyramidal neurons (Gould et al., 1997). Equally interesting would be to elucidate how antidepressants might prevent such stress-elicited morphological changes (Czeh et al., 2001). At this point it seems premature to proclaim that depression is associated with neuronal cell loss in the brain caused by stress hormones and that antidepressants work through remediation of this detrimental event through neurotrophin increase. In fact, Müller et al. (2002) showed that neither glucocorticoid treatment nor depression affect cellular integrity of the hippocampus, which is also in line with a study by Lucassen et al. (2001) rejecting hippocampal apoptosis associated with glucocorticoid overexposure.

Neurotensin (NT) — a mediator of antipsychotic-like symptoms

Since it was originally formulated by Arvid Carlsson the dopamine (DA) hypothesis of schizophrenia suggesting overactivity of mesolimbic DA system, remained the mainstay of schizophrenia research. This hypothesis has gained wide support since most effective antipsychotic drugs act through blockade of DA receptors, while drugs that enhance DA neurotransmission (including L-DOPA for the treatment of M. Parkinson) can produce psychotic symptoms. As discussed for affective disorders neuropeptides may also have a role in modulating monoamine transmitter actions which can lead to cardinal symptoms of schizophrenia. In this context NT, a tridecapeptide has been implicated in the pathogenesis of schizophrenia (review: Binder et al., 2001a).

CSF studies have consistently reported decreased NT content among schizophrenics and some but not all studies claimed that a successful antipsychotic treatment is associated with increased CSF NT concentration. There was a marked dissociation between CSF and plasma NT levels indicating that CSF NT levels reflect CNS extracellular fluid concentration and that NT in CSF is not derived from systemic circulation. Numerous post mortem studies were conducted which failed to produce clear results regarding different NT tissue concentrations in brains of schizophrenics and controls. Many behavioral and electrophysiological studies compared the effects of typical and atypical antipsychotic drugs with those of NT and found that the actions of the neuropeptide closely resemble those of atypical antipsychotics. Moreover, all clinically effective antipsychotic drugs increase NT mRNA and peptide concentration in the nucleus accumbens, a central brain region strongly implicated in the pathogenesis of schizophrenia (review: Binder et al., 2001a).

In dissecting the importance of NT in the pathogenesis and therapy of schizophrenia, studies which measured behavioral changes thought to model such psychophysiologic disturbances which are frequent in schizophrenia are of particular interest. A prevalent feature is a deficit in sensorimotor gating which prevents a schizophrenic patient from internal screening of sensory input, thus leading to an involuntary flooding of indifferent sensory data. This lack of gating and sorting of input possibly accounts for cognitive fragmentation and incoherent thought (Freedman et al., 1991).

One such psychophysiologic model is latent inhibition (review: Swerdlow and Geyer, 1998), which has been shown to have face, predictive and construct validity as an animal model for deficient sensorimotor gating in schizophrenic patients (Swerdlow et al., 1999). In fact, most studies agree that latent inhibition is enhanced by antipsychotic drugs. In contrast, NT receptor antagonists (SR 48692 or SR 142948A) dose dependently block latent inhibition in rats, pointing to a role for NT agonists as potential antipsychotics (Binder et al., 2002). In addition, the latent inhibition-enhancing effects of haloperidol (a typical antipsychotic drug) are blocked by pretreatment with a NT receptor antagonist (Binder et al., 2001b). Similarly the effects of typical and atypical antipsychotic drugs in another model of disrupted sensorimotor gating, deficient prepulse inhibition of the acoustic startle reflex in isolation reared rats, are also blocked by an NT receptor antagonist (Binder, 2001b). Interestingly, isolation reared rats also present with decreased NT mRNA and NT peptide concentrations in the nucleus accumbens, which are restored to normal by antipsychotic drug treatment (Binder et al., 2001b). In all, behavioral studies indicate that enhanced NT neurotransmission is apparently involved in the behavioral component of antipsychotic drug action and that NT agonist may serve a potential antipsychotic drugs. It has to be noted though that peripherally administered NT antagonists can also produce similar electrophysiological effects on DA neurons as atypical antipsychotic drugs (Binder et al., 2001a for review). To date, however, no behavioral effects for NT antagonists are reported that would reflect the central pharmacological findings.

Neuropeptides and sleep

The hypothalamic-pituitary adrenocortical system

One of the key behavioral response to a stressful situation is the lacking desire to fall asleep. As addressed above the major coordinator of behavioral adaptation to stress in the CNS is CRH. A study which administered CRH in a pulsatile mode, thus mimicking the naturally occurring secretion pattern identified a role for CRH as a neuropeptide that is also involved in sleep modulation of humans. Specifically, intravenous administration of 4 boluses of 50 μg CRH to normal male controls reduced slow wave sleep (the sleep stage believed to have profound recuperative effects) during the second half of the sleeping period as well as rapid eye movement (REM) sleep. In addition, the nocturnal secretion of growth hormone (which surges following sleep induction) was reduced (Holsboer et al., 1988). This finding was in line with a study where CRH was centrally administered to rats (Ehlers et al., 1986) and a confirmative study in humans (Tsuchiyama et al., 1995). The postulate that stress-elicited CRH inhibits sleep can be challenged by administration of CRH receptor antagonists (review: Holsboer, 1999). Studies using non-selective CRH receptor antagonists such as α-helical ovine$_{9-41}$(αh-CRH) and astressin — a CRH modified analog of D-Phe CRH$_{12-41}$ (Gulyas et al., 1995) — have so far reported conflicting results. A study by Chang and Opp (1998) applied centrally αh-CRH to rats at dark onset and observed a reduced amount of time spent awake during the first hours following drug administration. Astressin produced the same effect but with a long delay. When these compounds were administered at the beginning of the light period which coincides with the rest phase of these species, they failed to affect wakefulness which supports the view that CRH contributes to the regulation of physiological waking periods. In contrast, a study by Gonzales and Valatx (1998) found the opposite as these investigators failed to observe any effect of αh-CRH given at dark-onset upon sleep-wake behavior. Instead, αh-CRH abolished the increase in REM sleep normally induced by immobilization stress. Moreover, αh-CRH also reduced the rebound of REM sleep but not that of non-REM sleep usually following sleep-deprivation. One possible reason for these discrepancies is the absence of innate liability for increased stress response. Therefore, the rat strains generated by Rainer Landgraf displaying either increased (HAB rats) or decreased (LAB rats) anxiety-like behavior (see above) seem to be particularly suited to study the effects induced by blockade of CRH/CRHR1 signalling (review: Landgraf, 2001). Lancel et al. (2002) studied the sleep-EEG of these two rat lines and found that HAB rats spent less time in wakefulness and more time in nonREM sleep. When chemically stressed with a citrate buffer HAB rats showed a more profound stress response, i.e. they had higher plasma ACTH and corticosterone concentrations than LAB rats. Likewise, the effect of stress upon sleep was more vigorous among HAB rats which spent more time awake and less in nonREM sleep and had a longer latency to nonREM sleep in combination with fewer nonREM episodes. These stress-elicited sleep disturbances were prevented by R121919.

Specifically, addition of R121919 to the buffer solvent decreased circulating levels of ACTH and corticosterone, promoted nonREM sleep and REM sleep and increased slow wave activity in the EEG within nonREM sleep. Among LAB rats these sleep-EEG and neuroendocrine changes were less pronounced which accords with findings by Keck et al. (2001a) who found anxiolytic effects of R121919 in HAB rats only. Since these rats overproduce vasopressin in the hypothalamus it is interesting to note that acute vasopressin administration produces increased duration of waking, while a vasopressin antagonist produced the opposite effect (Arnauld et al., 1989). In contrast, in a study in elderly humans administration of vasopressin increased sleep period time and time spent in slow wave sleep and decreased the amount of REM sleep (Born et al., 1992; Perras et al., 1997). Taken together, it seems plausible to suggest that selective CRHR1 receptor antagonists have beneficial effects upon stress-related (depression associated) sleep disturbances (Held et al., unpublished) while vasopressin receptor antagonists do not seem to have effects in the same direction.

The somatotrophic system

The nocturnal growth hormone surge coincides with initiation of sleep and is timely associated with slow wave sleep suggesting a common physiological regulation (Steiger et al., 1987). Among depressives nocturnal growth hormone (GH)-release is blunted possibly due to increased CRH which when experimentally administered suppresses GH-secretion during sleep also in normal men (Holsboer et al., 1988). Steiger et al. (1992) administered growth hormone releasing hormone (GHRH) to young normal controls and found increased slow wave sleep. This study and a number of other studies corroborating the initial finding all agree that GHRH is a sleep promoting compound. Based on their studies with rats Ehlers and Kupfer (1987) submitted the possibility that a reciprocal interaction between GHRH and CRH might exist. This would be in line with the observations that CRH increases cortisol and suppresses GH and slow wave sleep, while GHRH infusion acts opposite increasing GH and slow wave sleep but decreasing cortisol secretion (see Fig. 5). The view that GHRH is an inducer of SWS is also corroborated by sleep-EEG studies in subjects with dwarfism due to lack of GHRH. These patients have decreased slow wave sleep (Aström and Lindholm, 1990). In contrast to GHRH, somatostatin which suppresses GH release was reported to decrease slow wave sleep, particularly in elderly patients (Frieboes et al., 1997). These data have quite convincingly demonstrated that clinical (e.g. depression) or physiological (increasing age) conditions associated with increased CRH and somatostatin secretion may be therapeutically counteracted by drugs that activate GHRH receptors (review: Steiger and Holsboer, 1997). A particularly exciting development stems from recent research with a novel peptide hormone isolated from stomach and hypothalamus and termed Ghrelin. This peptide binds to a recently cloned growth hormone (GH) secretagoge (S) receptor (GHS) to stimulate GH (review: Horvath et al., 2001). Thus, besides

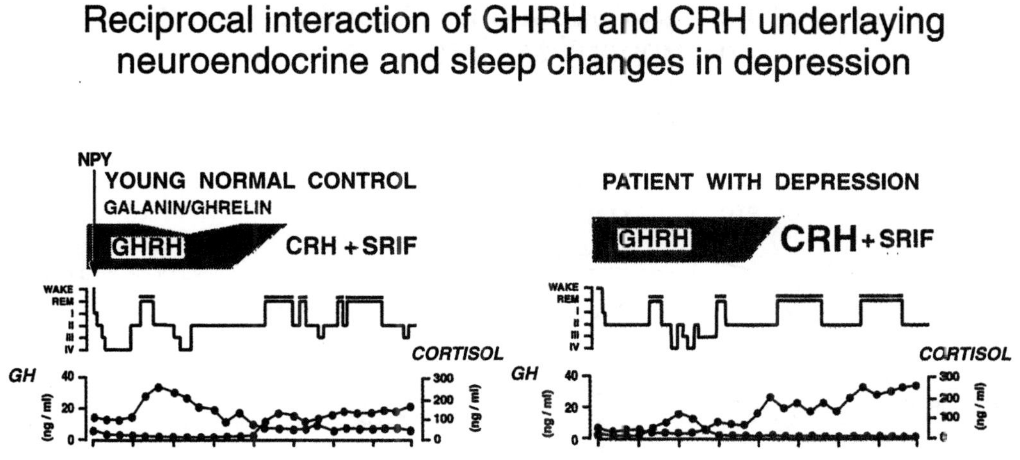

Fig. 5. Balance of hypothalamic growth hormone and corticotropin secretagogues in enhancement and suppression of sleep

GHRH another endogenous GH stimulant exists, challenging the hypothesis that GH secretagoges are somnogenic. The group by Axel Steiger recently showed that Ghrelin indeed promotes slow wave sleep in young healthy males (Weikel et al., unpublished). These preliminary data again point to a physiological role in the regulation of sleep in humans.

Conclusion and outlook

The few examples discussed in this treatise show that neuropeptides are important modulators of physiological and pathological effects in the brain. Neuropeptides are particularly suited as intervention targets as they are more likely to be hypersecreted under pathological conditions than amino acid or monoamine neurotransmitters. To illustrate: A CRHR1 antagonist has only effects if a pathological condition exists, i.e. a continuous stressor or innate high anxiety (Keck and Holsboer, 2001). In contrast, a modulator of $GABA_A$-channel such as a benzodiazepine has always effects ranging from anxiolysis to sedation and sleep induction depending on the pretreatment level of arousal. The use of peptides and proteins as drugs is limited because efficient delivery of proteins into cells in vivo can be achieved only when the molecules are small — typically less than 600 Daltons. Delivery of a peptide across the blood brain barrier is limited by the size (six amino acids or less) and the biochemical property (highly lipophilic) of the respective peptide. Although advocated by some, circumventing this problem by administering the peptides intranasally using the vomeronasal organ as a "leaky interface" does not resolve the issue as nerve cell delivery, i.e. passage through the cell membrane remains a problem except in cases where cell membrane receptors are to be targeted. The group by Dowdy has demonstrated that this problem can be overcome by

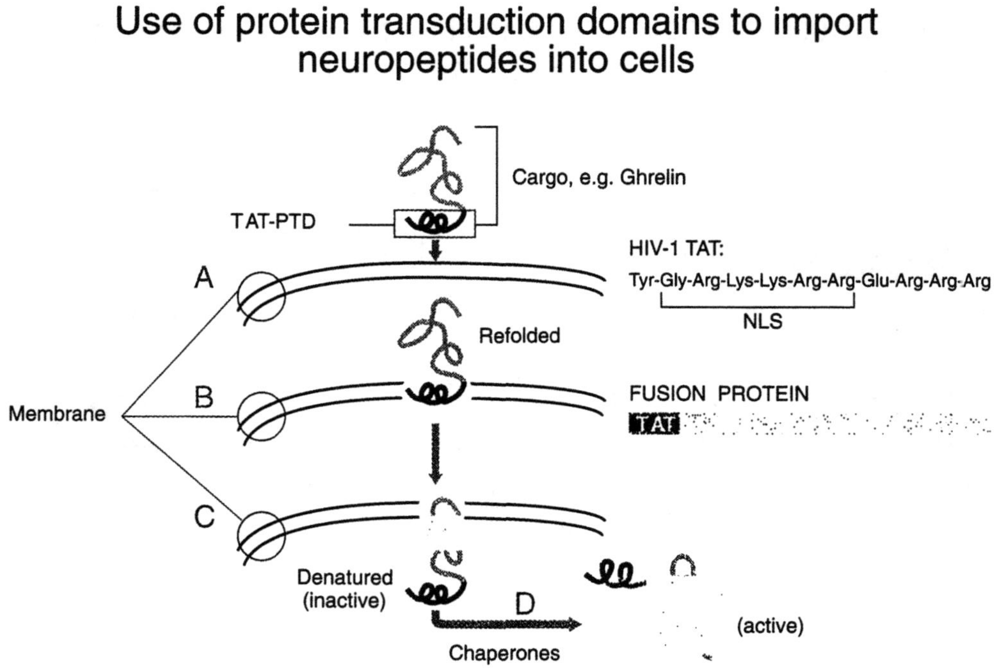

Fig. 6. Schematic representation of how linking a protein (cargo, e.g. Ghrelin) with a protein transduction domain (PTD) enables passage of a cargo protein (Ghrelin) through cell membranes (modified from Schwarze et al., 2000)

utilizing so-called protein transduction domains (review: Schwarze et al., 2000). These are amino acid sequences (10–16 residues long) which when fused to a protein, allow transduction through cell membranes in a receptor and transporter-independent fashion. These fusion proteins are capable to target the lipid bylayer directly. Thus, once a protein is identified as a potential drug target a fusion protein can be constructed that contains a protein transduction domain and interacts with the protein target (see Fig. 6). While this perspective is tempting it seems more realistic to use existing compound libraries and screen them with high throughput technology for orally available small molecules that pass the blood brain barrier and selectively interact with neuropeptides and their signalling cascades. It is beyond doubt that concerted efforts exploiting neuropeptide physiology in combination with functional genomics and proteomics as well as with medicinal chemistry will lead to drugs that are superior to the ones we currently use (Holsboer, 2001).

References

Arnauld E, Bibene V, Meynard J, Rodriguez F, Vincent JD (1989) Effects of chronic icv infusion of vasopressin on sleep-waking cycle of rats. Am J Physiol 256: R674–R684

Aström C, Lindholm J (1990) Growth hormone-deficient young adults have decreased deep sleep. Neuroendocrinology 51: 82–84

Bardeleben von U, Holsboer F (1991) Effect of age upon the cortisol response to human CRH in depressed patients pretreated with dexamethasone. Biol Psychiatry 29: 1042–1050

Bardeleben von U, Holsboer F, Stalla GK, Müller OA (1985) Combined administration of human corticotropin-releasing factor and lysine vasopressin induces cortisol escape from dexamethasone suppression in healthy subjects. Life Sci 37: 1613–1619

Binder EB, Kinkead B, Owens MJ, Nemeroff CB (2001a) The role of neurotensin in the pathophysiology of schizophrenia and the mechanism of action of antipsychotic drugs. Biol Psychiatry 50: 856–872

Binder EB, Kinkead B, Owens MJ, Kilts CD, Nemeroff CB (2001b) Enhanced neurotensin neurotransmission is involved in the clinically relevant behavioral effects of antipsychotic drugs: evidence from animal models of sensorimotor gating. J Neurosci 21: 601–608

Binder EB, Gross RE, Nemeroff CB, Kilts CD (2002) Effects of neurotensin receptor antagonism on latent inhibition in Sprague-Dawley rats. Psychopharmacology 161: 288–295

Born J, Kellner C, Uthgenannt D, Kern W, Fehm HL (1992) Vasopressin regulates human sleep by reducing rapid-eye-movement sleep. Am J Physiol 262: E295–E300

Bremner J, Narayan M, Anderson ER, Staib LH, Miller H, Charney DS (2000) Smaller hippocampal volume in major depression. Am J Psychiatry 157: 115–117

Chang FC, Opp MR (1998) Blockade of corticotropin-releasing hormone receptors reduces spontaneous waking in the rat. Am J Physiol 275: R793–R802

Chang L, Karin M (2001) Mammalian MAP kinase signalling cascades. Nature 410: 37–40

Chawla MK, Gutierrez GM, Young WS, McMullen NT, Rance NE (1997) Localization of neurons expressing substance P and neurokinin B gene transcripts in the human hypothalamus and basal forebrain. J Comp Neurol 384:429–442

Chen B, Dowlatshahi D, MacQueen GM, Wang JF, Young LT (2001) Increased hippocampal BDNF immunoreactivity in subjects treated with antidepressant medication. Biol Psychiatry 50: 260–265

Conti AC, Cryan JF, Dalvi A, Lucki I, Blendy JA (2002) cAMP response element-binding protein is essential for the upregulation of brain-derived neurotrophic factor transcription, but not the behavioral or endocrine responses to antidepressant drugs. J Neurosci 22: 3262–3268

Czeh B, Michaelis T, Watanabe T, Frahm J, de Biurrun G, van Kampen M, Bartolomucci A, Fuchs E (2001) Stress-induced changes in cerebral metabolites, hippocampal volume, and cell proliferation are prevented by antidepressant treatment with tianeptine. Proc Natl Acad Sci 98: 12796–12801

De Wied D (1993) From stress hormones to neuropeptides. In: Burbach JPH, de Wied D (eds) Brain functions of neuropeptides. A current view. The Parthenon Publishing Group, New York, pp 65–84

Dinan TG, Lavelle E, v. Scott L, Newell-Price J, Medbak S, Grossman AB (1999) Desmopressin normalizes the blunted adrenocorticotropin response to corticotropin-releasing hormone in melancholic depression: evidence of enhanced vasopressinergic responsitivity. J Clin Endocrinol Metab 84: 2238–2240

Dwivedi Y, Rizavi HS, Roberts RC, Conley RC, Tamminga CA, Pandey GN (2001) Reduced activation and expression of ERK1/2 MAP kinase in the post-mortem brain of depressed suicide subjects. J Neurochem 77: 916–928

Ehlers CL, Kupfer DJ (1987) Hypothalamic peptide modulation of EEG sleep in depression: a further application of the S-process hypothesis. Biol Psychiatry 22: 513–517

Ehlers CL, Reed TK, Henriksen SJ (1986) Effects of corticotropin-releasing factor and growth hormone-releasing factor on sleep and activity in rats. Neuroendocrinology 42: 467–474

File SE (2000) NKP608, an NK_1 receptor antagonist, has an anxiolytic action in the social interaction test in rats. Psychopharmacology 152: 105–109

Freedman R, Waldo M, Bickford-Wimer P, Nagamoto H (2001) Elementary neuronal dysfunctions in schizophrenia. Schizophr Res 4: 233–243

Frieboes RM, Murck H, Schier T, Holsboer F, Steiger A (1997) Somatostatin impairs sleep in elderly human subjects. Neuropsychopharmacology 16: 339–345

Gonzales MM, Valatx JL (1998) Involvement of stress in the sleep rebound mechanism induced by sleep deprivation in the rat: use of alpha-helical CRH (9–41). Behav Pharmacol 9: 655–662

Gould E, McEwen BS, Tanapat P, Galea LAM, Fuchs E (1997) Neurogenesis in the dentate gyrus of the adult tree shrew is regulated by psychosocial stress and NMDA receptor activation. J Neurosci 17: 2492–2498

Griebel G, Simiand J, Serradeil-LeGal C, Wagnon J, Pascal M, Scatton B, Maffrand JP, Soubrie P (2002) Anxiolytic- and antidepressant-like effects of the non-peptide vasopressin V_{1b} receptor antagonist, SSR149415, suggest an innovative approach for the treatment of stress-related disorders. Proc Natl Acad Sci Early Edition: 1–6

Gulyas J, Rivier C, Perrin M, Koerber SC, Sutton S, Corrigan A et al. (1995) Potent, structurally constrained agonists and competitive antagonists of corticotropin-releasing factor. Proc Natl Acad Sci 92: 10575–10579

Heuser I, Bissette G, Dettling M, Schweiger U, Gotthardt U, Schmider J, Lammers CH, Nemeroff CB, Holsboer F (1998) Cerebrospinal fluid concentrations of corticotropin-releasing hormone, vasopressin, and somatostatin in depressed patients and healthy controls: response to amitriptyline treatment. Depression & Anxiety 8: 71–79

Hökfelt T (1991) Neuropeptides in perspective: the last ten years. Neuron 7: 867–879

Holsboer F (1999) The rationale for corticotropin-releasing hormone receptor (CRH-R) antagonists to treat depression and anxiety. J Psychiatr Res 33: 181–214

Holsboer F (2000) The cortisol receptor hypothesis of depression. Neuropsychopharmacology 23: 477–501

Holsboer F (2001) Antidepressant drug discovery in the postgenomic era. World J Biol Psychiatry 2: 165–177

Holsboer F, Barden N (1996) Antidepressants and HPA regulation. Endcr Rev 17: 187–205

Holsboer F, von Bardeleben U, Steiger A (1988) Effects of intravenous corticotropin-releasing hormone upon sleep-related growth hormone surge and sleep EEG in man. Neuroendocrinology 48: 32–38

Horvath TL, Diano S, Sotonyi P, Heiman M, Tschöp M (2001) Ghrelin and the regulation of energy balance — a hypothalamic perspective. Endocrinology 142: 4163–4169

Hsu SY, Hsueh AJW (2001) Human stresscopin and stresscopin-related peptide are selective ligangs for the type 2 corticotropin-releasing hormone receptor. Nat Med 7: 605–611

Keck ME, Holsboer F (2001) Hyperactivity of CRH neuronal circuits as a target for therapeutic interventions in affective disorders. Peptides 22: 835–844

Keck ME, Welt T, Wigger A, Renner U, Engelmann M, Holsboer F, Landgraf R (2001a) The anxiolytic effect of the CRH_1 receptor antagonist R121919 depends on innate emotionality in rats. Eur J Neurosci 13: 373–380

Keck ME, Wigger A, Welt T, Müller MB, Gesing A, Reul JMHM, Holsboer F, Landgraf R, Neumann ID (2001b) Vasopressin mediates the response of the combined dexamethasone/CRH test in hyper-anxious rats: implications for pathogenesis of affective disorders. Neuropsychopharmacology 26: 94–105

Korte M, Carroll P, Wolf E, Brem G, Thoenen H, Bonhoeffer T (1995) Hippocampal long-term potentiation is impaired in mice lacking brain-derived neurotrophic factor. Proc Natl Acad Sci USA 92: 8.856–8.860

Kovalchuk Y, Hanse E, Kafitz KW, Konnerth A (2002) Postsynaptic induction of BDNF-mediated long-term potentiation. Science 295: 1729–1734

Kramer MS, Cutler N, Feighner J, Shrivastava R, Carman J et al. (1998) Distinct mechanism for antidepressant activity by blockade of central substance P receptors. Science 281: 1640–1645

Krieger DT (1983) Brain peptides: what, where and why? Science 222: 975–985
Lancel M, Müller-Preuss P, Wigger A, Landgraf R, Holsboer F (2002) The CRH1 receptor antagonist R121919 attenuates stress-elicited sleep disturbances in rats, particularly in those with high innate anxiety. J Psychiatr Res 36: 197–208
Landgraf R (2001) Neuropeptides and anxiety-related behavior. Endocr J 48: 517–533
Landgraf R, Gerstberger R, Montkowski A, Probst JC, Wotjak CT, Holsboer F, Engelmann M (1995) V1 vasopressin receptor antisense oligodeoxynucleotide into septum reduces vasopressin binding, social discrimination abilities, and anxiety-related behavior in rats. J Neurosci 15: 4250–4258
Liebsch G, Montkowski A, Holsboer F, Landgraf R (1998) Behavioral profiles of two Wistar rat lines selectively bred for high or low anxiety-related behavior. Behav Brain Res 94: 301–310
Linthorst ACE, Flachskamm C, Müller-Preuss P, Holsboer F, Reul JMHM (1995) Effect of bacterial endotoxin and interleukin-1β on hippocampal serotonergic neurotransmission, behavioral activity, and free corticosterone levels: an in vivo microdialysis study. J Neurosci 15: 2920–2934
Lucassen PJ, Müller MB, Holsboer F, Bauer J, Holtrop A, Wouda J, WJG Hoogendijk, De Kloet ER, Swaab DF (2001) Hippocampal apoptosis in major depression is a minor event and absent from subareas at risk for glucocorticoid overexposure. Am J Pathol 158: 453–468
Montkowski A, Holsboer F (1997) Intact spatial learning and memory in transgenic mice with reduced BDNE. Neuroreport 8: 779–782
Müller MB, Lucassen P, Yassouridis A, Hoogendijk WGJ, Holsboer F, Swaab DF (2001) Neither major depression nor glucocorticoid treatment affects the cellular integrity of the human hippocampus. Eur J Neurosci 14: 1603–1612
Müller MB, Preil J, Renner U, Zimmermann S, Kresse AE, Stalla GK, Keck ME, Holsboer F, Wurst W (2001) Expression of CRHR1 and CRHR2 in mouse pituitary and adrenal gland: implications for HPA system regulation. Endocrinology 142: 4150–4153
Nibuya M, Takahashi M, Russel DS, Duman RS (1999) Chronic stress increases catalytic TrB mRNA in rat hippocampus. Neurosci Lett 267: 81–84
Penalva RG, Flachskamm C, Zimmermann S, Wurst W, Holsboer F, Reul JMHM, Linthorst ACE (2002) Corticotropin-releasing hormone receptor type 1-deficiency enhances hippocampal serotonergic neurotransmission: an in vivo microdialysis study in mutant mice. Neuroscience 109: 253–266
Perras B, Pannenborg H, Marshall L, Pietrowsky R, Born J, Fehm HL (1997) Three months of intranasal vasopressin increased sleep time, slow wave sleep and REM sleep in healthy old humans. Exp Clin Endocrinol Diabetes [Suppl] 1: 23
Preil J, Müller MB, Gesing A, Reul JMHM, Sillaber I, Gaalen M, Landgrebe J, Stenzel-Poore M, Holsboer F, Wurst W (2001) Regulation of the hypothalamic-pituitary-adrenocortical system in mice deficient for corticotropin-releasing hormone receptor 1 and 2. Endocrinology 142: 4946–4955
Purba JS, Hoogendijk WJG, Hofman MA, Swaab DF (1996) Increased number of vasopressin- and oxytocin-expressing neurons in the paraventricular nucleus of the hypothalamus in depression. Arch Gen Psychiatry 53: 137–143
Raadsheer FC, Hoogendijk WJG, Stam FC, Tilders FHJ, Swaab DF (1994) Increased numbers of corticotropin-releasing hormone expressing neurons in the hypothalamic paraventricular nucleus of depressed patients. Neuroendocrinology 60: 433–436
Reul JMHM, Holsboer F (2002) Corticotropin-releasing factor receptors 1 and 2 in anxiety and depression. Curr Opin Pharmacol 2: 23–33
Santarelli L, Gobbi G, Debs PC, Sibille EL, Blier P, Hen R, Heath MJS (2001) Genetic and pharmacological disruption of neurokinin 1 receptor function decreases anxiety-related behaviors and increases serotonergic function. Proc Natl Acad Sci USA 98: 1912–1917

Schwarze SR, Hruska KA, Dowdy SF (2000) Protein transduction: unrestricted delivery into all cells? Trends Cell Biol 10: 290–295
Sheline Y, Wany P, Gado MH, Csernansky JG, Vannier MW (1996) Hippocampal atrophy in recurrent major depression. Proc Natl Acad Sci USA 93: 3908–3913
Sheline Y, Sanghavi M, Mintun MA, Gado MH (1999) Depression duration but not age predicts hippocampal volume loss in medically healthy women with recurrent major depression. J Neurosci 19: 5034–5043
Shirayama Y, Chen ACH, Nakagawa S, Russel DS, Duman RS (2002) Brain-derived neurotrophic factor produces antidepressant effects in behavioral models of depression. J Neurosci 22: 3251–3261
Sillaber I, Rammes G, Zimmermann S, Mahal B, Zieglgänsberger W, Wurst W, Holsboer F, Spanagel R (2002) Enhanced and delayed stress-induced alcohol drinking in mice lacking functional CRH1 receptors. Science 296: 931–933
Smith MA, Makino S, Kvetnansky R, Post RM (1995) Stress alters the express of brain-derived neurotrophic factor and neurotrophin-3 mR-NAs in the hippocampus. J Neurosci 15: 1768–1777
Spengler D, Rupprecht R, Phi Van L, Holsboer F (1992) Identification and characterization of a 3′,5′-cyclic adenosine monophosphate-responsive element in the human corticotropin-releasing hormone gene promoter. Mol Endocrinol 6: 1931–1941
Steiger A, Holsboer F (1997) Neuropeptides and human sleep. Sleep 20: 1038–1052
Steiger A, Herth T, Holsboer F (1987) Sleep-electroencephalography and the secretion of cortisol and growth hormone in normal controls. Acta Endocrinol (Copenh) 116: 36–42
Steiger A, Guldner J, Hemmeter U, Rothe B, Wiedemann K, Holsboer F (1992) Effects of growth hormone-releasing hormone and somatostatin on sleep EEG and nocturnal hormone secretion in male controls. Neuroendocrinology 56: 566–573
Swerdlow NR, Geyer MA (1998) Using an animal model of deficient sensorimotor gating to study the pathophysiology and new treatments of schizophrenia. Schizophr Bull 24: 285–301
Swerdlow NR, Braff DL, Geyer MA (1999) Cross-species studies of sensorimotor gating of the startle reflex. Ann NY Acad Sci 877: 202–216
Teixeira RM, Santos AR, Ribeiro SJ, Calixto JB, Rae GA, De Lima TC (1996) Effects of central administration of tachykinin receptor agonists and antagonists on plus-maze behavior in mice. Eur J Pharmacol 311: 7–14
Thome J, Sakai N, Shin K, Steffen C, Zhang YJ, Impey S, Storm D, Duman RS (2000) Cyclic AMP response element-mediated gene transcription is upregulated by chronic antidepressant treatment. J Neurosci 20: 4030–4036
Timpl P, Spanagel R, Sillaber I, Kresse A, Reul JMHM, Stalla GK, Blanquet V, Steckler T, Holsboer F, Wurst W (1998) Impaired stress response adn reduced anxiety in mice lacking a functional corticotropin-releasing hormone receptor 1. Nat Genet 19: 162–166
Tsuchiyama Y, Uchimura N, Sakamoto T, Maeda H, Kotorii T (1995) Effects of hCRH on sleep and body temperature rhythms. Psychiatry Clin Neurosci 49: 299–304
Zobel AW, Nickel T, Künzel HE, Ackl N, Sonntag A, Ising M, Holsboer F (2000) Effects of the high-affinity corticotropin-releasing hormone receptor 1 antagonist R121919 in major depression: the first 20 patients treated. J Psychiatr Res 34: 171–181

Authors' address: Prof. F. Holsboer, MD, PhD, Max Planck Institute of Psychiatry, Kraepelinstrasse 2-10, D-80804 Munich, Federal Republic of Germany, e-mail: holsboer@mpipsykl.mpg.de

J Neural Transm (2003) [Suppl] 64: 35–63

Pharmacological approaches to migraine

H.-Ch. Diener

Department of Neurology, University Essen, Federal Republic of Germany

Summary. Migraine is a paroxysmal disorder with attacks of headache, nausea, vomiting, photo- and phonophobia and malaise. This review summarises new treatment options both for the therapy of the acute attack as well as for migraine prophylaxis. Analgesics like aspirin or nonsteroidal antiinflammatory drugs (NSAIDs) are effective in treating migraine attacks. Few controlled trials were perfomed for the use of ergotamine or dihydroergotamine. These trials indicate inferior efficacy compared to serotonin $(5\text{-HT})_{1B/D}$-agonists (further on called "triptans"). The triptans (almotriptan, eletriptan, frovatriptan, naratriptan, rizatriptan, sumatriptan and zolmitriptan) are highly effective. They improve headache as well as nausea, photo- and phonophobia. The different triptans have minor differences in efficacy, headache recurrence and adverse effects. The knowledge of their different pharmacological profile allows a more specific treatment of the individual migraine characteristics. Migraine prophylaxis is recommended, when more than 3 attacks occur per month, if attacks do not respond to acute treatment or if side effects of acute treatment are severe. Substances with proven efficacy include the beta-blockers metoprolol and propranolol, the calcium channel blocker flunarizine, several 5-HT antagonists and amitriptyline. Recently antiepileptic drugs (valproic acid, gabapentin, topiramate) were evaluated for the prophylaxis of migraine. The use of botulinum-toxin is under investigation.

Introduction

This review focusses on the new class of $5\text{-HT}_{1B/D}$-agonists and some other new approaches towards the treatment of acute migraine attacks and migraine prophylaxis. Studies with oral and s.c. sumatriptan were summarized some years ago by Tfelt-Hansen [1]. We will summarize new information on the pharmacology of the new migraine drugs and report the results from clinical trials. A comparison between anti-migraine drugs is only possible in randomized controlled trials (RCTs) with head-to-head comparisons. When these are not available, indirect although less reliable information can be gained by comparing net therapeutic gain. Therapeutic gain is the difference in efficacy between active drug and placebo [2]. Another way to indirectly compare the different triptans is a metaanlysis [3]. The primary endpoint in most headache trials is the improvement from severe or moderate head pain to mild or no pain after 120 minutes. The most recent recommendations of the International Headache Society, however, propose 2 hour pain free and 24 hours sustained pain free (pain free after 2 hours, no rescue medication, no recurrence) as the appropriate endpoints for clinical trials in migraine treatment [4]. Readers who want a comprehensive review on the epidemiology, genetics, clinic and pathophysiology of migraine are refered to the articles by Goadsby et al. [5].

Sumatriptan

The most comprehensive review about the efficacy and adverse events of 6 mg subcutaneous, 100 mg oral and 20 mg intranasal sumatriptan was written by Tfelt-Hansen [6]. He calculated numbers needed to treat (NNT) which is the number of patients needed to be treated in the active drug group in order to obtain relief which would not have been obtained with placebo and numbers needed to harm (NNH) to evaluate side effects. Twelve RCTs were performed with 100 mg oral sumatriptan. The success rate was 58% (1067/1854) for sumatriptan compared to 25% (256/1036) for placebo resulting in a NNT of 3.0 (95% CI 2.8–3.4) and NNH of 8.3 (95% CI 6.3–12.2). For subcutaneous sumatriptan 12 RCTs were available. The success rate of sumatriptan after 1 hour was 69% (1337/1927) and of placebo 19% (226/1200) resulting in a NNT of 2.0 (1.9–2.1) and a NNH of 3.0 (2.7–3.4). Finally 6 trials were performed with intranasal sumatriptan and a success rate after 2 hours of 61% (563/917) compared to placebo 30% (149/503) and NNT of 3.1 (2.7–3.8) was achieved. These data clearly indicate, that subcutaneous sumatriptan is the most effective treatment but causes more side effects than oral sumatriptan. In a large dose-finding trial 50 mg and 100 mg oral sumatriptan were equally effective and superior to 25 mg sumatriptan. The 50 mg dose had fewer side effects than the higher dose and therefore is the preferred initial dose [7].

Following more than 80 international trials of oral and subcutaneous sumatriptan [8, 9], sumatriptan was developed in intranasal and suppository formulations for patients unable to take tablets and unwilling to inject themselves. In the intranasal formulation sumatriptan has a T-max of 1 h (subcutaneously 0.2 h, orally 1.5 h) and a half-life of 2 hours [10]. In a dose-finding study (n = 544) dosages of 2.5, 5, 10 and 20 mg were compared [11]. Dosages of 5, 10 and 20 mg reduced the headache within 2 hours significantly in 49%, 46% and 64% of the patients, respectively. Two additional trials comparing 10 mg and 20 mg with placebo (n = 409 and 436) showed a significant relief of headache within 2 hours in 43–54% of the patients receiving the 10 mg dose and in 62–63% receiving 20 mg compared to 29–35% with placebo [12]. A retrospective analysis of four pooled trials performed between 1993 and 1994 including 2395 patients [13] showed no influence of sex, age, migraine type (with or without aura), weight, pretreatment headache duration and migraine prophylaxis on the success rates. In a multiple attack treatment trial two thirds of the patients treating 3 attacks with 20 mg sumatriptan nasal spray experienced relief at 2 hours postdose in at least 2 of 3 attacks [14]. In addition to the known side effects taste disturbances were the only side effects reported [15]. The approved doses for the nasal spray are 10 and 20mg.

Sumatriptan as a suppository was tested in a double-blind placebo-controlled trial including 431 patients with dosages of 6, 12.5, 25, 50, and 100mg. Dosages of 12.5mg and upwards showed a significant improvement of headache within 2 hours. However, there were no statistical differences between these dosages. Two hours following the drug administration 65%, 72%, 66% and 70% of the patients reported significant improvement of headache receiving 12.5, 25, 50 and 100mg, respectively [16]. A randomised double-blind, parallel-group, placebo controlled trial in 184 patients compared 12.5mg, 25mg sumatriptan suppositories with placebo. Relief rates 2 hours post-dose were 68% in the high dose group, 47% with 12.5mg and 25% with placebo [17]. The approved dose of the sumatriptan suppository is 25mg.

One study investigated the use of sumatriptan in children and found no difference between active drug and placebo [18]. This is most probably due to the fact, that migraine attacks have a short duration in children and therefore seem to respond well to placebo. In addition children have a much higher placebo response. Überall and Wenzel performed a study with 20mg intranasal sumatriptan in children with long lasting attacks not responding to conventional therapy with analgesics or ergots [19]. Under these conditions sumatriptan was superior to placebo.

Pharmacokinetic and clinical studies revealed no interaction of sumatriptan with DHE, butorphanol, naratriptan or drugs used for migraine prophylaxis such as propranolol, flunarizine, pizotifen, paroxetine and fluoxetine [9, 20]. Systemic sumatriptan exposure is increased in patients who are treated with monoamine oxidase inhibitors (MAOI). One study, however treated 28 patients who were on MAOI's with 6mg sumatriptan and found no increase in adverse events but observed a lower recurrence rate [21].

All triptans have vasoconstrictive action and are contraindicated in patients with vascular disease. Postmarketing surveillance studies and case reports indicate, that sumatriptan, albeit rarely, is associated with serious cardiovascular events including myocardial infarction [22–25], cardiac arrythmia [26], stroke [27–29] and ischemic colitis [30]. The frequency of serious adverse events is about 1:1 million treated attacks [31, 32]. Almost all serious adverse events occurred in patients with contraindications or other diseases than migraine. A positron emission tomography study in healthy volunteers showed, that 6mg sumatriptan s.c. has no influence on myocardial perfusion [33]. GlaxoSmithKline established a pregnancy register to obtain data from patients and newborns when sumatriptan was taken during pregnancy (although not recommended). Up to now the data from almost 300 pregnancies are available and indicate that there is no increased risk of major birth defects [34, 35]. Two other observational studies found no increase in fetal malformations [36, 37].

The next "triptans" (Table 1)

Following sumatriptan, several new 5-HT$_{1B/D}$-agonists have been developed and introduced in the last few years. The further development of new 5-HT$_{1B/D}$-agonists was motivated by the intention to improve the pharmacological and pharmacokinetic properties of sumatriptan. Sumatriptan has a poor oral bioavailability (14%) and and a low penetration of the blood-brain barrier. The low penetration, however, seems not to affect the efficacy of sumatriptan. This could indicate, that the blood-brain barrier becomes leaky during a migraine attack. Most of the new drugs have already been studied extensively in clinical trials. Almotriptan, frovatriptan, eletriptan, naratriptan, rizatriptan and zolmitriptan have finished phase III clinical trials and are approved in most countries. The further development of alniditan [38] was halted due to a lack of improvement against sumatriptan and avitriptan [39, 40] due to hepatic side effects. Donitriptan just entered phase II trials [41].

Table 1. Therapy of acute migraine attacks in the adult

Substance	Dose (mg)	Indication	Side effects	Contraindications
Sumatriptan (***)	25–100 PO 25 PR 20 IN 6 SC	Moderate or severe headache Severe headache, early vomiting and diarhoea	Warmth sensation, fatigue, dizziness, chest tightness	Vascular disease, MI, coronary heart disease, stroke, TIA, multiple vascular risk factors
Almotriptan (***)	12.5 PO	See sumatriptan	Fewer than sumatriptan	As for sumatriptan
Frovatriptan (**)	2.5 PO	Moderate headache	Fewer than sumatriptan	As for sumatriptan
Eletriptan (***)	20, 40, 80 PO	See sumatriptan	See sumatriptan	As for sumatriptan
Naratriptan (***)	2.5 PO	Moderate headache	chest tightness, warmth sensation, tingling	As for sumatriptan
Rizatriptan (***)	5 or 10 PO	Moderate or severe headache	like sumatriptan	As for sumatriptan
Zolmitriptan (***)	2.5–5 PO	Moderate or severe headache	Asthenia, somnolence, dizziness chest tightness	As for sumatriptan

*** Treatment recommendations based on more than one well-designed randomized, placebo-controlled trial or a metaanlysis; ** Treatment is based on least one randomized prospective study of reasonable size; * Treatment based on personal experience, expert opinion, retrospective or nonrandomised studies. *PO* oral; *PR* rectal, suppository; *IV* intravenous; *IM* intramuscular, *IN* intranasal

Naratriptan

Naratriptan has a better pharmacokinetic profile than sumatriptan: the bioavailability of the oral formulation is almost 60% (sumatriptan = 14%) which reduces the effective dosage to 2.5 mg. Moreover, the half-life is about 5 hours, 2–3 times longer than the half-life of oral sumatriptan, which may account for a reduced percentage of patients with headache recurrence in some studies [42, 43]. However, possibly due to a higher affinity for the 5-$HT_{1B/D}$-receptor, the vasoconstrictive activity in animal experiments was higher than that of sumatriptan [44]. Therefore naratriptan at the moment is only available in oral form. Dose-finding trials with doses of naratriptan between 0.1 and 10 mg showed the best relationship between efficacy and side effects to be at doses of 2.5 mg [42, 43, 45]. Publications initially reported only 4 hour efficacy data, which indicated a slow onset of action. Goadsby [46] and Salonen [47] had access to 2 hour data and calculated NNT for naratriptan 2.5 mg of 4.8 compared with 3.0 for 50 and 100 mg oral sumatriptan. An interesting aspect is, that naratriptan given subcutaneously is at least as effective as s.c. sumatriptan and has a linear dose-efficacy relationship [48]. The low dose of oral naratriptan was chosen based on tolerability. At an oral dose of 2.5 mg naratriptan has an favourable side effect profile and is undistinguishable from placebo [49]. 1 mg naratriptan is available in the USA. Subcutaneous naratriptan (not available for treatment) in dosages of 1, 2.5 and 5 mg caused an increase in mean peak systolic blood pressure of 8, 15 and 15 mmHg, respectively, when compared with placebo [50]. Naratriptan has a low recurrence rate after initial efficacy [51]. It should be noted, however, that recurrence can only occur in patients who initially have a positive response to a headache drug. Naratriptan should be used in patients with moderate migraine attacks who are unable to tolerate the side effects of oral sumatriptan.

Zolmitriptan

Zolmitripan was the second triptan to enter the market. The pharmacokinetic profile offers interesting improvements compared to oral sumatriptan. With an oral bioavailability of almost 50% (sumatriptan 14%) the neccessary clinical effective dosage could be significantly reduced. In addition to its vascular effects zolmitriptan has a central mode of action [52]. Zolmitriptan has been evaluated over a wide range of doses (1–25 mg). and has shown a consistently high headache response rate across placebo-controlled trials [53–56]. The decision was made to market the oral 2.5 mg dose. Headache response rate for this dose at 2 hours was 62% (N = 219) compared to 36% for placebo (N = 108) [57]. The rate of pain free response after 2 hours across all dose-finding studies was 25% (N = 438) [58]. The rate of headache recurrence (27–33%) was comparable to that of sumatriptan. One placebo-controlled study compared zolmitriptan 5 mg with sumatriptan 100 mg [56]. This study employed an unusual skewed randomisation ratio (1:8:8) for placebo, zolmitriptan and sumatriptan. Due to the small number of patients in the placebo group resulting in large confidence intervals, no difference was seen between the 3 treatment groups in terms of the primary endpoint e.g. complete headache response. In a long-term safety and efficacy trial including more than 2200 patients with over 20.000 migraine attacks using 5 mg of oral zolmitriptan, neither safety nor efficacy were affected when the drug was used in up to 30 consecutive attacks [59]. Zolmitriptan nasal spray (5 mg) has a higher efficacy than oral application and an earlier onset of action [60]. The 2 hour response rate of the 5 mg spray was 70% compared to 30% with placebo [61]. In contrast to sumatriptan, nasal zolmitriptan is absorbed via the nasal mucosa [62]. Side effects and CNS adverse events of oral zolmitriptan are similar to those of oral sumatriptan, although zolmitriptan can cross the blood-brain barrier [63]. Zolmitriptan has no interactions with dihydroergotamine, ergotamine, pizotifen, fluoxetine, paracetamol, or selegeline [64]. Coadministration of propranolol resulted in a 56% increase in the area under the plasma concentration-time curve of zolmitriptan [65]. With a dose of 2.5 mg zolmitriptan no additional side effects were seen when combining it with propranolol. MAO-A inhibitors (moclobemide) result in increased plasma levels of zolmitriptan and its metabolites. Therefore it would be prudent to limit the total daily dose should several doses be required [64]. In clinical practice, 2.5 mg zolmitriptan is at least equivalent to 50 mg sumatriptan. In some patients who do not respond to sumatriptan zolmitriptan is effective and vice versa. 5 mg zolmitriptan is equivalent to 100 mg sumatriptan. Some patients who do not respond to 2.5 mg zolmitriptan will show a response to the 5 mg dose.

Rizatriptan

Rizatriptan also has an improved pharmacokinetic profile. The oral bioavailability of rizatriptan is about 40% versus 14% for oral sumatriptan. Rizatriptan's T_{max} is 1 hour versus 2.5 hours for oral sumatriptan, suggesting the potential for a faster onset of action in favor of rizatriptan. The half-life, however, is about 3 hours. Two clinical dose-finding studies have been carried out including 865 patients. Dosages were tested between 2.5–40 mg. The first study compared 10, 20 and 40 mg with 100 mg sumatriptan and placebo [66] and the second trial 2.5, 5 and 10 mg with placebo [67]. Dosages of 5 mg and above were effective, with 10 mg being the most effective dosage with reasonable side effects. Two hours following the administration of the drug 21%, 47%, 52%, 56% and 64% of the patients reported relief from headache receiving 2.5, 5, 10, 20 and 40 mg rizatriptan, respectively (placebo 18%, sumatriptan 100 mg 46%). In a large placebo-controlled trial (N = 1473) rizatritpan 10 mg had a success rate of 71%, rizatriptan 5 mg 62% and placebo 35% [68]. Two placebo-controlled studies compared rizatriptan to oral sumatriptan and found that rizatriptan 10 mg had earlier onset of headache relief than sumatriptan 100 and 50 mg [69, 70]. Rizatriptan 10 mg was also superior to sumatriptan 100 mg on pain-free response and reduction in functional disability. Rizatriptan 10 mg has also demonstrated consistent response across four migraine attacks [71]. Of the 252 patients who treated 3 attacks with rizatriptan, 96%, 86%, and 60% reported relief from headache at 2 hours in 1 out of 3, 2 out of 3, and 3 out of 3 attacks, respectively. In another comparative trial the efficacy of zolmitriptan and rizatriptan was identical for the 2 hour headache response [72]. Concerning the endpoints time to pain free and pain free after 2 hours, rizatriptan was superior to zolmitriptan. Rizatriptan was clearly superior to naratriptan [73, 74]. Fourty-five percent of patients were pain free 2 hours after intake of 10 mg rizatriptan (n = 201) compared to 21% with 2.5 mg naratriptan (n = 213) and 8% with placebo (n = 107).

In addition to oral tablets, rizatriptan is available in a wafer which dissolves instantly on the tongue without liquid. Trial results with this application form indicate that the efficacy is comparable compared to the tablet, but that patients prefer the wafer [75–77]. Side effects increased dose dependently and were typical for drugs of this class. Rizatriptan has an interaction with propranolol (not with metoprolol). Patients who are on propranolol prophylaxis for their migraine should only take rizatriptan 5 mg. Rizatriptan has comparable recurrence to oral sumatriptan [70]. In summary rizatriptan 10 mg has a slightly faster onset of action and is somewhat more effective than oral sumatriptan.

Eletriptan

Eletriptan has been approved recently in oral doses of 20 and 40. In some countries the 80 mg dose was also approved. Like the other new $5\text{-HT}_{1B/D}$-agonists, eletriptan has an improved oral bioavailability (almost 50%), is rapidly absorbed and has a half-life of 4–5 hours [78]. Two multicenter dose finding studies have been carried out to evaluate the clinical efficacy of the drug. In the first trial (n = 365) 5, 20 and 30 mg of oral eletriptan were tested in the treatment of acute migraine attacks. At 2 hours after treatment, significant relief of headache was reported by 41, 47 and 49% of the patients, respectively (placebo: 35%) [79]. In a second trial with 857 migraine patients 20, 40 and 80 mg of eletriptan were evaluated against 100 mg of sumatriptan and placebo. Headache response two hours following the administration of the drug could be observed in 55%, 65%, 77% and 56% of the patients receiving 20, 40, and 80 mg of eletriptan or sumatriptan 100 mg, respectively (placebo: 24%) [80, 81]. One should note, however, that sumatriptan was encapsulated in the comparative trials which might have affected absorption. The rate of adverse events in the group receiving 80 mg eletriptan was higher compared with the rate in the group receiving 100 mg sumatriptan. In all other treatment groups the rate of adverse events was significantly lower. The most recent trial [81] compared 40 mg eletriptan (n = 452) with 80 mg (n = 461) and placebo (n = 238). Headache relief after 2 hours was reported by 62% and 65% of the patients in the active treatment goups and 19% of those patients on placebo. Of those patients with a headache response at 2 hours after 80 mg eletriptan 21% had a headache recurrence after a mean time of 19 hours. In an other comparative trial 40 and 80 mg eletriptan were significantly better effective than Cafergot (2 mg ergotamine plus 200 mg caffeine) [82].

Almotriptan

In dose-finding studies 2, 6.25, 12.5 und 25 mg almotriptan were compared to placebo. Almotriptan was superior to placebo from a dose of 6.25 mg on. Headache response after 2 hours was 58.5% with 12.5 mg almotriptan compared to 32.5% with placebo. The pain free rates after 2 hours were 38% with 12.5 mg almotriptan and 11% with placebo [83, 84]. In another placebo-controlled trial with 722 patients 6.25 and 12.5 mg almotriptan were used to treat 3 consecutive migraine attacks [85]. Efficacy after 2 hours was 38% for placebo, 60% for 6.25 mg almotriptan und 70% for 12,5 mg almotriptan. Efficacy in 2 out of 3 migraine attacks was 64% for the lower and 75% for the higher dose. Headache recurrence was identical in the 3 treated attacks and ranged between 28.7 and 30.1% for the two almotriptan doses. Another comparative trial compared 12.5 and 25 mg almotriptan and 100 mg sumatriptan. The efficacy of sumatriptan and almotriptan was identical [86]. Almotriptan had fewer side effects. Pascual performed a meta-analysis oif 2294 patients treated with almotriptan [84]. The efficacy of 12.5 mg almotriptan after 2 hours was 64% compared to placebo (35%). The numbers for pain free after 2 hours were 36% versus 14%. In another comparative trial including 1173 patients with 50 mg sumatriptan, almotriptan showed identical efficacy with the exception of the 2 hour pain free rate which was higher for sumatriptan [87]. Long-term trials showed sustained efficacy, few adverse events and a low number of drop-outs due to adverse events [88, 89].

Frovatriptan

Frovatriptan has an interesting receptor profile. The compound has a higher affinity to $5HT_{1B/1D}$ — receptors than sumatriptan, but is an agonist of $5HT_7$ receptors as well [90]. This is interesting because activation of $5HT_7$ receptors (in higher dosages) might cause vasodilatation e.g. on coronary vessels (possibly indicating no cardio-vascular side effects due to vasoconstriction). In oral dose finding studies (1–100 mg), dosages of 2.5 mg and dosages above were effective [91, 92]. The pharmacokinetic properties however, are similar to those of naratriptan: the drug is relatively slowly absorbed and reaches its T_{max} after 2 hours. The most relevant parameter to measure efficacy of a migraine drug is the percentage of patients who are pain free after 2 hours [93]. This measure is robust (patients have no difficulty to judge whether they have pain or not) and has a low placebo rate (<10%). Results for pain free are 15% for 2.5 mg frovatriptan compared to 5% with placebo resulting in a therapeutic gain of 10% only. The second best outcome parameter is improvement of headache from servere or moderate to mild or no headache, the so called "Glaxo" criteria [94]. The efficacy rate for frovatriptan 2.5 mg is between 38 and 42%. Since their are no direct comparative trials with other triptans (except sumatriptan) an indirect way to compare triptans is by way of therapeutic gain [95]. Therapeutic gain for 2.5 mg frovatriptan ranges from 15% to 26% compared to 33% for sumatriptan (100 mg), 22% for naratriptan (2.5 mg), 29% for zolmitriptan (2.5 mg), 36% for rizatriptan (10 mg) and 42% for eletriptan (40 mg) [96]. Frovatiriptan therefore ranges at the low end of efficacy. Four hour data are less important, since patients want a fast onset of action. The rate of headache recurrence varies between 25% and 40% for the other triptans. Lowest recurrence rates have been reported for naratriptan (25%) and eletriptan 80 mg (24%). One has to keep in mind, that recurrence only can occur after initial improvement of headache. Therefore drugs with a low efficacy such as naratriptan and frovatriptan also will have a low recurrence rate. The only way to get around this problem is to report sustained pain free data: pain free after 2 hours, no recurrence for the next 24 hours and no intake of rescue medication. These data were not yet reported for frovatriptan. One claim of the manufacturer of frovatriptan is its improved cardiac safety. For the other triptans, severe cardiac events are reported at a rate of 1–500.000 to 1:1 million treated migraine attacks [32]. Therefore this claim can only be made when more than 50 million migraine attacks were treated with frovatriptan. One should keep in mind that tolerability is assessed in phase II and III trials, but not safety which requires postmarketing surveys in large numbers of patients. In summary, frovatriptan offers no advantages over the other triptans.

The triptan meta-analysis

Ferrari et al. (3) performed a meta-analysis of 53 triptan trials, 12 of which were not yet published. The analysis is based on data from 24.089 patients. Endpoints for the analysis were headache response (improvement of headache from severe or moderate to mild or no headache) 2 hours after intake of study medication and pain free response. Other endpoints were headache recurrence and consistency in 2 out of 3 treated migraine attacks. Studies were included if they were randomised, double-blind and compared one triptan to placebo or another triptan. Oral sumatriptan 100 mg was taken as the reference drug. 59% of patients had a headache response after 2 hours and 29% were pain free. Sustained pain free, which means pain free after 2 hours, no recurrence and no intake of rescue medication were 20% of patients. Consistency was 67%. Sumatriptan 50 mg is as effective as the 100 mg dose, but has fewer side effects. Rizatriptan 10 mg is more effective than 100 mg sumatriptan, but has a higher recurrence rate. Rizatriptan has the best consistency. Naratriptan and frovatriptan are less effective than sumatriptan. Zolmitriptan 2.5 and 5 mg are as effective as sumatriptan and have a similar side effect profile. Eletriptan is available in doses of 20 and 40 mg and in some countries in a 80 mg dose. 20 mg are inferior to sumatriptan and 40 mg are equivalent. Eletriptan 80 is more effective than sumatriptan, has a lower recurrence rate but more side effects. Almotriptan 12.5 mg is as effective as sumatriptan for headache response and seems to be superior for pain free. This, however, is not longer the case, when therapeutic gain is calculated. Almotriptan has a good side effect profile.

Problems with triptans

Even the new 5-$HT_{1B/D}$-agonists will not solve the problems of this class of substances. Despite improved pharmacokinetics and -dynamics, up to 40% of all attacks and up to 25% of all patients do not respond to any of these substances. It is unclear whether the "non-responders" have a variant of migraine or a different 5-HT receptor profile. Some patients may suffer from tension-type headache with migraine features and are likely to not respond to a triptan. If a patient with migraine does not respond to a particular triptan on three attacks it is worthwhile to try another triptan [97]. If a patient does not respond to three oral triptans, s.c. sumatriptan should be tested. If this also is not effective the patient is either a "triptan-nonreponder" or does not suffer from migraine. Most 5-$HT_{1B/D}$-agonists have a ceiling effect where higher doses do not lead to improved efficacy. Eletriptan is the exception. 20, 40 and 80 mg have a linear dose-efficacy relationship. Longer half-lifes of new migraine drugs were supposed to decrease headache recurrence [98]. This has not been the case, as drugs with longer half-lifes than sumatriptan also show headache recurrence, although with a slightly longer time interval [92, 99].

Another problem is the likelihood that all new 5-$HT_{1B/D}$-agonists taken too often, will decrease the time interval between migraine attacks, which results in medication-overuse headache such as has been observed in conjunction with ergotamine, DHE and sumatriptan [100–106]. A recent population-based study in Denmark indicates that a small number of patients uses sumatriptan on a daily or almost daily basis [103]. Whether these patients had chronic cluster headache or were abusing sumatriptan is not known. We observed recently medication overuse headache after use of zolmitriptan and naratriptan [106]. Of this group five patients using zolmitriptan only (who had never taken ergotamine derivatives or other triptans before) developed drug induced headache after a period of six month only, partly with a dosage of only 7.5 mg a week (only 3 tablets weekly). This indicates that second-generation triptans with their improved pharmacological profile cause drug induced chronic daily headache faster and at lower dosages than expected or that a pronounced central effect of action is supporting the development of drug induced chronic daily headache. Finally, all 5-$HT_{1B/D}$ agonists have vasoconstrictive activity. Using human coronary arteries there was no difference, the vasoconstriction was almost identical between the triptans [107, 108].

New developments

Some recent studies indicated, that triptans might be more effective when taken early in the attack as long as the headache is mild [109]. Patients should only be advised to take a triptan early if they only suffer from migraine and not from migraine and tension-type headache and only if they have few attacks per month. Otherwise, the intake of triptans may beome to frequent, leading to medication overuse headache.

Other new drugs for the treatment of migraine attacks

Apart from the new 5-$HT_{1B/D}$-agonists several other classes of drugs have been suggested as potentially beneficial in the acute treatment of migraine. Since substance P is known to play a crucial role in the transmission of nociception, neurokinin (NK)-antagonists have received special interest as potential analgesics. In several animal models of neurogenic inflammation, NK-antagonists have been shown to attenuate nociceptive impulses. In an international multicenter trial an oral preparation of the NK-antagonist RPR 100893 was evaluated in the acute treatment of migraine. Unfortunately the drug did not perform better than placebo [110]. The trial, however, suffered from poor design. Trials with other NK antagonists (LY 303870) were also negative [111].

Another group of drugs that may be of potential benefit in migraine treatment are endothelin-antagonists. An international multicenter trial evaluated an intravenous form of the endothelin antagonist bosentan in the acute treatment of migraine, but the drug did not perform better than placebo [112]. Recently, Lassen and Olesen [113] presented preliminary data of the nitric oxid synthese inhibitor 546 C 88. In a pilot study including 15 patients and 10 controls using an intravenous formulation, 8 patients reported a significant relief from headache. Further clinical trials will be neccessary to confirm these data.

New approaches include substances that modulate ion-channels. LY293558 is an AMPA/KA receptor antagonist and given iv is effective in the treatment of migraine attacks [114]. GLUR5 antagonists and adenosine A_1 receptor agonists are still at the level of animal experiments. Lilly developed a highly selective 5-HT_{1F}-agonist-without vasoconstrictive properties [115]. The results from clinical trials in acute migraine showed efficacy [116]. The further development of the drug was interrupted until it will become clear whether it has hepatic side effects.

Additional new classes of drugs are currently being tested (e.g. 5-HT_{1F}-agonists and CGRP-antagonists). Hence, it seems reasonable to predict that in the future we will have a wide range of new drugs which will enable us to successfully treat the vast majority of our headache patients with a minimum of side effects.

Analgesics and non-steroidal antiinflammatory drugs

Many OTC drugs for the treatment of pain and headache contain more than one compound. These "mixtures" were mostly based on assumptions and not on sound clinical trials. Recently three placebo controlled studies were performed in 1357 patients with migraine [117]. Patients with moderate to severe headache (not requiring bed rest) took either 2 tablets of active drug containing 250 mg paracetamol (acetaminophen), 250 mg aspirin and 65 mg caffeine or placebo. Pain relief after 2 hours was achieved by 59% of patients in the active group and by 33% in the placebo group. Comparisons with triptans are impossible, since these studies were biased towards patients with moderate attacks. The most critical question remained unanswered, namely, whether an adequte dose of a monosubstance (e.g. 1,000 mg aspirin) would achieve the same goal. Myllylä et al. [118] treated 2 migraine attacks in 140 patients either with 200 mg rapid-release tolfenamic acid or 100 mg sumatiptan. The two active treatment groups showed no significant difference for headache relief after 2 hours (tolfenanim acid; attack 1 77%, attack 2 70%, sumatriptan; attack 1 79%, attack 2 64%), but both were different from placebo (attack 1 29%, attack 2 39%). This result together with the positive result from an older trial in which 1680 mg oral lysine acetylsalicylate (= 1000 mg aspirin) plus 10 mg metoclopramide were as effective as sumatriptan [119] justifies in de novo patients and countries with limited drug budgets the so called step-care approach. Patients are first treated with analgesics plus metoclopramide or an ergot plus an antiemetic (Table 2). Ergots are mentioned because they are cheap, not because they offer an alternative for the triptans. If this treatment fails or results in adverse events, only than will the treatment proceed to the triptans. Ibuprofen 200 mg is as effective as 400 mg and superior to placebo [120]. Diclofenac potassium is more rapidly absorbed than normal diclofenac. 50 and 100 mg diclofenac potassium are as effective as 100 mg sumatriptan sodium and superior to placebo [121–123].

Conclusion

The triptans were a major step forward, both in the understanding of head pain in migraine and in the therapy of acute migraine attacks. There is, however, still place for improvement in terms of efficacy, headache recurrence and side effects.

Preventative treatment

The prophylactic treatment of migraine is an appealing therapeutic approach. The ideal drug or procedure would completely abolish migraine attacks, resolving patient's symptoms. To date, this goal has been unattainable, with few drugs being more than 50% effective and with patients still requiring acute treatment.

The mode of action for most drugs used in migraine prophylaxis is not known and animal models to test the action of drugs used for migraine prophylaxis are not available. A powerful placebo effect exists [124, 125], which can lead to a decrease in migraine frequency of up to 70% within

Table 2. Therapy of acute migraine attacks in the adults

Substance	Dose (mg), route	Indication	Side effects	Contraindications
I. Antiemetics				
Metoclopramide (**)	10–20 PO 20 PR 10 IV, IM	improves nausea and vomiting, absorption of analgesics	extrapyramidal system oculogyric crisis (treatment biperidin i.v.)	children <12 years
Domperidone (*)	10–20 PO	As for metoclopramide	As for metoclopramide	As for metoclopramide
II. Analgesics				
1. Acetylsalicylic acid (***)	500–1000 PO as effervescent tablet	moderate headache	gastric pain bronchospasm hemorrhages tinnitus	GI ulcer Asthma
Lysine acetylsalicylate (***)	500–1000 IV	Moderate and severe headache	As for ASA	As for ASA
2. Paracetamol (**)	500–1000 PO, PR	moderate headache		liver disease
3. Ibuprofen (**)	100–400 PO	moderate headache	As for ASA	As for ASA
4. Diclofenac-K	50–100 PO	Moderate and severe headache	As for ASA	As for ASA
III. Others				
1. Ergotamine (**)	2 PO, PR; max per attack = 4 mg; max per month = 16 mg	severe headache	nausea, vomiting, tightness of the chest, headache	peripheral artery disease, coronary heart disease, hypertension
2. Dihydro-ergotamine (DHE) (***)	1 SC or IV; not sufficiently absorbed orally	severe headache	As for ergotamine	As for ergotamine

PO oral; *PR* rectal, suppository; *IV* intravenous; *IM* intramuscular; symbols see Table 1

Table 3. Migraine prophylaxis: effective substances in the order of therapeutic choice. First choice: Beta-receptor-blockers

Substance	Dose/day	Remarks/Mechanism of action
Metoprolol (***)	initially 50; later 150–200 mg	beta-1-selective
Propranolol (***)	initially 40; later 160–200 mg	non selective

*** Treatment recommendations based on more than one well-designed randomized, placebo-controlled trial or a metaanlysis; ** Treatment is based on least one randomized prospective study of reasonable size; * Treatment based on personal experience, expert opinion, retrospective or nonrandomised studies

3 months [126, 127]. Couch [128] analysed some parallel and double-blind studies on the prevention of migraine. The effect of placebo in the reduction of frequency and severity of migraine attacks ranged from 11 to 36%. This effect decreased after 3 months. It is still not known whether prophylaxis is more effective using a combination of drugs rather than monotherapy. However, it is preferable to avoid combinations of drugs because, in such instances, adverse effects are more frequent than with monotherapy and sometimes cannot be attributed to a single substance.

The different spectrum of adverse effects is another problem in patients with migraine pain. Clinical experience shows, that adverse-effects are more frequent in patients with migraine than in those taking the same drugs for other reasons. Compliance with migraine prophylaxis can below. One of the reasons is, that patients first experience adverse effects and only with a delay od weeks any beneficial effect of the drug. The following part focus on the most important aspects of migraine prophylaxis and the different compounds are considered in the order of their efficacy and risk-benefit ratio.

Beta-adrenoceptor antagonists

Prophylactic of migraine headache by beta-blockers was detected incidentally in patients who were treated for hypertension or angina pectoris and who also suffered from migraine headaches [129]. Propranolol [130, 131] and metoprolol [132–134] have both been convincingly shown to have migraine prophylactic activity. This was shown in placebo-controlled trials and in comparative trials against flunarizine, pizotifen and methysergide [135–143]. Administration, adverse effects and contraindications for propranolol and metoprolol are listed in Table 3. Atenolol [144, 145], timolol [146–148], nadolol [149] and bisoprolol [138, 150, 151] are beta-blockers with a possible prophylactic action. No migraine prophylactic activity has been shown for acebutolol, alprenolol, oxprenolol and pindolol [152]. Holroyd et al. performed a meta-analysis for propranolol in the prophylaxis of migraine [130]. The 53 studies included in the meta-analysis reported 2,403 patients who were treated with either the beta-blocker (propranolol 160 mg) or a reference substance or placebo. On average, propranolol yielded a 44% reduction in

Table 4. Migraine prophylaxis. Second choice: Calcium-antagonists and valproic acid

Substance	Dose/day	Remarks/Mechanism of action
Flunarizine (***)	initially 5 mg; later 10 mg in man, 5 mg in women	long half-life; calcium-channel antagonist and 5-HT antagonist
Valproic acid (***)	500–600 mg	GABAergic acting drug

migraine activity when daily headache recordings were used to assess treatment outcome, and a 65% reduction of migraine activity when clinical ratings of improvement and global patient reports were used. The drop-out rate due to side effects was 5.3%.

Calcium channel blockers

Flunarizine was introduced as a calcium-antagonist for the prophylaxis of migraine on the hypothetical basis of being protective against brain hypoxia. It has, however, a large spectrum of side effects: antidopaminergic (extrapyramidal motor system), antiserotonergic (sedation, weight gain) and antinoradrenergic (depression) properties (Table 4). Flunarizine is not approved in all countries for migraine prophylaxis despite the fact that it has shown its efficacy in many controlled trials [153]. Pure calcium antagonists like verapamil are either only marginally effective [154, 155] or as in the cases of nifedipine [156, 157] and nimodipine [126, 127] are ineffective. Verapamil is used in countries were flunarizine is not available. Cyclandelate is another calcium channel blocker which was recently investigated for migraine prophylaxis with different results. In a large recently conducted multicenter trial the substance was not superior to placebo [158].

Dihydroergotamine (DHE)

DHE is still widely used as a prophylactic medication in some European countries, but has been poorly studied using modern double-blind or placebo-controlled techniques [159, 160]. DHE was significantly more effective than placebo in reducing the frequency of migraine attacks. It should, however, be kept in mind that the prolonged use of DHE can lead to chronic daily headache.

Serotonin receptor antagonists

Methysergide and pizotifen (Table 5) are thought to act as 5-HT_2 antagonists. Both substances are clearly effective, but have a high frequency of adverse

Table 5. Migraine prophyalxis. Third choice: ASA, NSAIDs and Serotonin-antagonists

Substance	Dose/day	Remarks/Mechanism of action
Acetylsalicylic acid (**)	300 mg	inhibitor of prostaglandin synthesis
Naproxen (**)	3 × 250 mg	inhibitor of prostaglandin synthesis
Methysergide (***)	2–8 mg	not >6 months (retroperitoneal fibrosis) Serotonin-antagonist (5-HT2)
Pizotifen (**)	3 × 0.5 mg	Serotonin-antagonist (5-HT2)
Alpha-dihydro-ergocryptine (*)	1 × 10 mg	Dopamine-agonist
Lisuride (*)	3 × 0.025 mg	Dopamine-agonist

effects [161]. Methysergide can (rarely) lead to retroperitoneal fibrosis and therefore should not be given for longer than 6 months. It raises the mean blood pressure and constricts peripheral vessel (e.g. coronary arteries) and is therefore contraindicated in patients with cardio-vascular risk factors. Further adverse events are sedation, dizziness and weight gain. Few cases of of cardiac valvular lesions have been reported with the use of methysergide. Its use should now be restricted to patients with cluster-headache and to migraine patients who do not respond to other prophylactics. Pizotifen does not lead to retroperitoneal fibrosis, but shows the same profile of adverse events like methysergide and is be a drug of third choice as well.

Aspirin and NSAIDs

NSAIDs and ASA are well established in the acute treatment of migraine attacks. The first indications that the regular intake of ASA could act as a migraine prophylaxis came from the Physicians' Health study [162]. This study investigated the use of 325 mg ASA (every 2nd day) versus placebo in 22,071 male physicians for the prevention of myocardial infarction and stroke. ASA resulted in a 20% reduction of migraine attacks in the 661 men with migraine. In a controlled study with cross-over design, Grotemeyer et al. [163] compared 200 mg metoprolol and ASA 1,500 mg per day. A significant reduction in migraine frequency could be observed in 67% of the patients in the metoprolol group compared with only 14% in the ASA group. A recent study compared 300 mg aspirin with 200 mg metoprolol in 270 migraine patients. Aspirin was less effective (responder rate 42.7% versus 56.9%) compared to metoprolol, but had fewer side effects [164]. Low dose aspirin was not effective in a large placebo-controlled trial in women [165]. Naproxen sodium is established in migraine prophylaxis as well (Table 5, [166–169]). Studies indicate that naproxen is as effective as pizotifen and can be used for the prophylaxis of menstrual migraine [170]. Other NSAIDs like ketoprofen, mefenamic acid, tolfenamic acid and lornoxicam are also effective but the number of controlled trials is much smaller than for naproxen [171–173]. The clinical experience, however, shows that some patients with migraine do not tolerate NSAIDs for a longer time due to their gastro-intestinal adverse effects.

Other prophylactic treatments

Lisuride is approved in some countries for the prophylaxis of migraine (Table 5). Its action is probably mediated through dopamine- and 5-HT-receptors. Amitriptyline has been used in only a few controlled trials [174–176]. Its efficacy in migraine prophylaxis is low, though it can be recommended in selected patients with a combination of tension-type headache and infrequent migraine attacks. It is more popular in the USA, where many prophylactic agents used in other countries are not available. Selective serotonin reuptake inhibitors are not effective in migraine prophylaxis. Dopamine agonists like alpha-DHEC are probably effective [177]. High dose magnesium has shown conflicting results. One placebo controlled trial in patients from private practice found a positive effect on migraine frequency [178], while another study in patients from headache centers was unable to replicate this result [179]. In one open and one placebo-controlled trial 400 mg riboflavin (vitamin B2) were effective in the prophylaxis of migraine [180, 181]. The reduction in migraine frequency was between 60 and 70%. The possible role of injections of low doses of botulinum toxin in pericranial and cervical muscles is under investigation [182].

Antiepileptic drugs

Recent studies indicate that valproic acid has a prophylactic value in migraine [183–187]. Valproic acid reduces the frequency of migraine attacks, but not their severity and duration of attacks. Doses as low as 500–600 mg/day seem to be as effective as higher doses. Lamotrigine is not effective in migraine prophylaxis [188]. In some patients with migraine with aura it showed some efficacy [189]. In a recent placebo-controlled trial, gabapentin was superior to placebo in migraine prophylaxis [190]. Topiramate was effective in small open trials [191–194]. Three major placebo-controlled trials and one trial in comparison with propranolol are underway at present.

Prophylaxis of menstrual migraine

Prophylaxis is necessary whenever acute migraine attacks during menstruation cannot be treated with success. First, oral contraceptives should be stopped. As second choice beta-blockers or flunarizine can be used. Prophylaxis may sometimes be achieved by naproxen 250 mg twice daily given 4 days before until 3 days after menstruation. An open pilot study described a prophylactic action of 25 mg sumatriptan tid taken 2–3 days prior to menstrua-

Table 6. Special populations in migraine prophylaxis

Clinical situation	Treatment options
Menstrually-related headache	NSAIDs with cycle Ergotamine po nocte Oestrogen patches Low dose sumatriptan
Children (<12 yrs)	Betablockers Low dose DHE
Elderly (>65 yrs)	Beta-blockers in patients with hypertension

tion [195]. Naratriptan 1 mg bid, but not 2.5 mg were effective in the prevention of menstrual migraine in a placebo-controlled trial [196]. Estrogen given as patch transdermal therapeutic systems (TTS 100) is also effective in the prevention of menstrual migraine [197].

Prophylaxis of pediatric headache

There are few controlled trials of migraine prophylaxis in children. Drugs include beta-blockers, low dose flunarizine (5 mg/day), low doses of amitriptyline (1 mg/kg/body wheight) [198] or DHE 1–2 mg/day [199]. Behavioral therapy is the treatment of choice in children.

Prophylaxis in the elderly

In elderly patients without heart block, diabetes or asthma the drugs of first choice are beta — blockers (Table 6). Flunarizine may lead to hyokinesia, rigidity and tremor and 5-HT-anatgonists can induce depressions. Valproic acid is well tolerated in the elderly, but dose increases should be performed more slowly than in younger people.

Future prospects

The treatment of acute migraine attacks, despite the progress by the introduction of the triptans is far from perfect. There is still a need for more effective drugs with a higher consistency. Effective drugs without vasoconstrictive properties are needed to treat migraine patients with vascular diseases and vascular risk factors. Headache recurrence ist still a major problem. Idealy a drug for the treatment of a migraine attack should terminate the attack and not only improve the symptoms for a limited time. More progress is needed in the prevention of migraine. There still is no animal model for migraine prophylaxis. There are no trials investigating which biological variables or characteristics of migraine would predict efficacy or failure of a particular substance for migraine prophylaxis. Combination therapy is used in many fields of neurology, e.g. Parkinsons disease, epilepsy and stroke prevention. Combination therapy for the prevention of migraine was never properly studied. This would be an important approach to therapy for the upcoming years.

References

1. Tfelt-Hansen P (1996) Drug treatment of migraine: acute treatment and migraine prophylaxis. Curr Opin Neurol 9: 211–213
2. Tfelt-Hansen P (1997) Preliminary analysis of randomized placebo-controlled clinical trials with newer 5-HT1D receptor agonists for the treatment of migraine attacks. In: Olesen J, Tfelt-Hansen P (eds) Headache treatment: trial methodology and new drugs, vol 6. Lippincott-Raven, New York, pp 253–256
3. Ferrari MD, Roon KI, Lipton RB, Goadsby PJ (2001) Oral triptans (serotonin 5-$HT_{1B/1D}$ agonists) in acute migraine treatment: a meta-analysis of 53 trials. Lancet 358: 1668–1675
4. Tfelt-Hansen P, Block G, Dahlof C, Diener HC, Ferrari MD, Goadsby PJ, Guidetti V, Jones B, Lipton RB, Massiou H, Meinert C, Sandrini G, Steiner T, Winter PB, for the International Headache Society Clinical Trials Subcommittee (2000) Guidelines for controlled trials of drugs in migraine: second edition. Cephalalgia 20: 765–786
5. Goadsby PJ, Lipton RB, Ferrari MD (2002) Migraine — current understanding and treatment. N Engl J Med 346: 257–270
6. Tfelt-Hansen P (1998) Efficacy and adverse events of subcutaneous, oral, and intranasal sumatriptan used for migraine treatment: a systematic review based on numbers needed to treat. Cephalalgia 18: 532–538
7. Pfaffenrath V, Cunin G, Sjonell G, Prendergast S (1998) Efficacy and safety of sumatriptan tablets (25 mg, 50 mg, and 100 mg) in the acute treatment of migraine: defining the optimum doses of oral sumatriptan. Headache 38: 184–190
8. Wilkinson M, Pfaffenrath V, Schoenen J, Diener HC, Steiner T (1995) Migraine and cluster headache — their management with sumatriptan: a critical review of the current clinical experience. Cephalalgia 15: 337–357
9. Perry CM, Markham A (1998) Sumatriptan. An updated review of its use in migraine. Drugs 55: 889–922
10. Moore K, Hussey E, Shaw S, Fuseau E, Duquesnoy C, Pakes G (1997) Safety, tolerability and pharmacokinetics of sumatriptan in healthy subjects following ascending intranasal doses and multiple intransal doses. Cephalalgia 17: 541–550
11. Becker WJ, on behalf of the Study Group (1995) A placebo-controlled, dose-defining study of sumatriptan nasal spray in the acute treatment of migraine. Cephalalgia 15[Suppl 14]: 271–276
12. Ryan R, Elkind A, Baker CC, Mullican W, DeBussy S, Asgharnejad M (1997) Sumatriptan nasal spray for the acute treatment of migraine. Neurology 49: 1225–1230
13. Ashford E, Salonen R, Saiers J, Woessner M (1998) Consistency of response to sumatriptan nasal spray across patient subgroups and migraine types. Cephalalgia 18: 273–277
14. Diamond S, Elkind A, Jackson RT, Ryan R, DeBussey S, Asgharnejad M (1998) Multiple-attack efficacy and tolerability of sumatriptan nasal spray in the treatment of migraine. Arch Fam Med 7: 234–240
15. Diener HC (2000) Sumatriptan — Therapy. In: Diener HC (ed) Drug treatment of migraine and other headaches. Karger, Basel, pp 93–109

16. Göbel H, on behalf of the Study Group (1995) A placebo-controlled, dose defining study of sumatriptan suppositories in the acute treatment of migraine. Cephalalgia 15[Suppl 14]: 232
17. Tepper SJ, Cochran A, Hobbs S, Woessner M, on the behalf of the S2B351 Study Group (1998) Sumatriptan suppositories for the acute treatment of migraine. Int J Clin Pract 52: 31–35
18. Hämäläinen ML, Hoppu K, Santavuori P (1997) Sumatriptan for migraine attacks in children: A randomized placebo-controlled study. Do children with migraine attacks respond to oral sumatriptan differently from adults? Neurology 48: 1100–1103
19. Überall MA, Wenzel D (1999) Intranasal sumatriptan for the acute treatment of migraine in children. Neurology 52: 1507–1510
20. Joffe RT, Sokolov ST (1997) Co-administration of fluoxetine and sumatriptan: the Canadian experience. Acta Psychiatr Scand 95: 551–552
21. Freitag FG, Diamond S, Diamond M, Urban G, Pepper B (1998) Subcutaneous sumatriptan in patients treated with monoamine oxidase inhibitors and other prophylactic agents. Headache Quarterly 9: 165–171
22. O'Connor P, Gladstone P (1995) Oral sumatriptan-associated transmural myocardial infarction. Neurology 45: 2274–2276
23. Main ML, Ramaswamy K, Andrews TC (1998) Cardiac arrest and myocardial infarction immediately after sumatriptan injection (letter). Ann Intern Med 128: 874
24. Ottervanger JP, Paalman HJA, Boxma GL, Stricker BHC (1993) Transmural myocardial infarction with sumatriptan. Lancet 341: 861–862
25. Mueller L, Gallagher RM, Ciervo CA (1996) Vasospasm-induced myocardial infarction with sumatriptan. Headache 36: 329–331
26. Ottervanger JP, Stricker BHC (1995) Cardiovascular adverse reactions to sumatriptan — cause for concern? CNS Drugs 3: 90–98
27. Cavazos JE, Carees JB, Chilukuri VR (1994) Sumatriptan-induced stroke in sagittal sinus thrombosis. Lancet 343: 1105–1106
28. Luman W, Gray RS (1993) Adverse reactions associated with sumatriptan. Lancet 341: 1091–1092
29. Jayamaha JEL, Street MK (1995) Fatal cerebellar infarction in a migraine sufferer whilst receiving sumatriptan. Intensive Care Med 21: 82–83
30. Knudsen JF, Friedman B, Chen M, Goldwasser JE (1998) Ischemic colitis and sumatriptan use. Arch Intern Med 158: 1946–1948
31. Welch KMA, Mathew NT, Stone P, Rosamond W, Saiers J, Gutterman D (2000) Tolerability of sumatriptan: clinical trials and post-marketing experience. Cephalalgia 20: 687–695
32. O'Quinn S, Davis R, Guttermann D, Pait G, Fox A (1999) Prospective large-scale study of the tolerability of subcutaneous sumatriptan injection for the acute treatment of migraine. Cephalalgia 19: 223–231
33. Lewis PJ, Barrington SF, Marsden PK, Maisey MN, Lewis LD (1997) A study of the effects of sumatriptan on myocardial perfusion in healthy male migraineurs using 13NH3 positron emission tomography. Cephalalgia 48: 1542–1550
34. Shuhaiber S, Pastuszak A, Schick B, Matsui D, Spivey G, Brochu J, Koren G (1998) Pregnancy outcome following first trimester exposure to sumatriptan. Neurology 51: 581–583
35. Fox AW, Chambers CD, Anderson PO, Diamond ML, Spierings ELH (2002) Evidence-based assessment of pregnancy outcome after sumatriptan exposure. Headache 42: 8–15
36. Olesen C, Steffensen FH, Sorensen HT, Nielsen GL, Olsen J (2000) Pregnancy outcome following prescription for sumatriptan. Headache 40: 20–24
37. O'Quinn S, Ephross SA, Williams V, Davis RL, Gutterman DL, Fox AW (1999) Pregnancy and perinatal outcomes in migraineurs using sumatriptan: a prospective study. Arch Gynecol Obstet 263: 7–12

38. Goldstein J, Dahlöf CGH, Diener HC, Olesen J, Schellens R, Senard JM, Simard D, Steiner TJ, on behalf of the Subcutaneous Alniditan Study G (1996) Alniditan in the acute treatment of migraine attacks: a subcutaneous dose-finding study. Cephalalgia 16: 497–502
39. Couch JR, Saper J, Meloche JP, for the North American BMS Study Group (1996) Treatment of migraine with BMS 180048: response at 2 hours. Headache 36: 523–530
40. Ryan RE, Elkind A, Goldstein J (1997) Twenty-four-hour effictiveness of BMS 180048 in the acute treatment of migraine headaches. Headache 37: 245–248
41. John GW, Perez M, Pawels PJ, Le Grand B, Verscheure Y, Colpaert FC (2000) Donitriptan, a unique high efficacy 5-$HT_{1B/1D}$ agonist: key features and acute antimigraine potential. CNS Drug Rev 6: 278–289
42. Klassen A, Elkind A, Asharnejad M, Webster C, Laurenza A, on behalf of the Naratriptan S2WA3001 Study Group (1997) Naratriptan is effective and well tolerated in the acute treatment of migraine. Results of a double-blind, placebo-controlled, parallel-group study. Headache 37: 630–645
43. Mathew NT, Asgharnejad M, Peykamian M, Laurenza A, on behalf of the Naratriptan S2WA3001 Study Group (1997) Naratriptan is effective and well tolerated in the acute treatment of migraine. Results of a double-blind, placebo-controlled, crossover study. Neurology 49: 1485–1490
44. Connor HE, Feniuk W, Beattie DT, North PC, Oxford AW, Saynor DA, Humphrey PPA (1997) Naratriptan: biological profile in animal models relevant to migraine. Cephalalgia 17: 145–152
45. Gunasekara NS, Wiseman LR (1997) Naratriptan. CNS Drugs 8: 402–408
46. Goadsby PJ (1998) A triptan too far? J Neurol Neurosurg Psychiatry 64: 143–147
47. Salonen R (1999) Naratriptan. Int J Clin Pract 53: 552–556
48. Dahlöf C, Hogenhuis L, Olesen J, Petit H, Ribbat J, Schoenen J, Boswell D, Fuseau E, Hassani H, Winter P (1998) Early clinical experience with subcutaneous naratriptan in the acute treatment of migraine: a dose-ranging study. Eur J Neurol 5: 469–477
49. Heywood J, Bomhof MAM, Pradalier A, Thaventhiran L, Winter P, Hassani H (2000) Tolerability and efficacy of naratriptan tablets in the acute treatment of migraine attacks for 1 year. Cephalalgia 20: 470–474
50. Kempsford RD, Lacey LF, Keene ON (1993) The safety, tolerability and pharmacokinetics of subcutaneous GR 85548, a novel 5-HT1-receptor agonist for the treatment of migraine. Br J Clin Pharmacol 36: 170
51. Sheftell F, O'Quinn S, Watson C, Pait D, Winter P (2000) Low migraine headache recurrence with naratriptan: clinical parameters related to recurrence. Headache 40: 103–110
52. Goadsby PJ, Knight YE (1997) Direct evidence for central sites of action of zolmitriptan (311C90): an autoradiographic study in cat. Cephalalgia 17: 153–158
53. Ferrari MD (1997) 311C90: Increasing the options for the therapy with effective acute antimigraine 5HT1B/D receptor agonists. Neurology 48[Suppl 3]: 21–24
54. Rapoport AM, Ramadan NM, Adelmann JU, Mathew NT, Elkind AH, Kudrow DB, Earl NL, on behalf of The 017 Clinical Trial Study Group (1997) Optimizing the dose of zolmitriptan (Zomig, 311C90) for the acute treatment of migraine. A multicenter, double-blind, placebo-controlled, dose-finding study. Neurology 49: 1210–1218
55. Dahlöf C, Diener HC, Goadsby PJ, Massiou H, Olesen J, Schoenen J, Wilkinson M, Sweet RM, Klein KB (1998) Zolmitriptan, a 5-HT1B/D receptor agonist for the acute oral treatment of migraine: a multicentre, dose-range finding study. Eur J Neurol 5: 535–543
56. Geraud G, Olesen J, Pfaffenrath V, Tfelt-Hansen P, Zupping R, Diener HC, Sweet R, on behalf of the Study Group (2000) Comparison of the efficacy of zolmitriptan and sumatriptan: issues in migraine trial design. Cephalalgia 20: 30–38

57. Solomon GD, Cade RK, Klapper JA, Earl NL, Saper JR, Ramadan NM, on behalf of The 042 Clinical Trial Study Group (1997) Clinical efficacy and tolerability of 2.5 mg zolmitriptan for the acute treatment of migraine. Neurology 49: 1219–1225
58. Schoenen J, Sawyer J (1997) Zolmitriptan (Zomig, 311C90), a novel dual central and peripheral 5HT1B/1D agonist: an overview of efficacy. Cephalalgia 17[Suppl 18]: 28–40
59. The International 311C90 Long-Term Study Group (1998) The long-term tolerability and efficacy of oral zolmitriptan (Zomig, 311C90) in the acute treatment of migraine. An international study. Headache 38: 173–183
60. Becker WJ, Lee D (2001) Zolmitriptan nasal spray is effective, fast-acting and well tolerated during both, short- and long-term treatment. Cephalalgia 21: 271
61. Dowson AJ, Boes-Hansen S, Farkkila AM (2000) Zolmitriptan nasal spray is fast-acting and highly effective in the acute treatment of migraine. Eur J Neurol 7[Suppl 3]: 82
62. Sorensen J, Bergstrom M, Antoni A, Nairn K, Yates R, Kemp J, Dane A (2000) Distribution of 11C-zolmitriptan nasal spray assessed by positron emission tomography (PET). Eur J Neurol 7[Suppl 3]: 82
63. Edmeads JG, Millson DS (1997) Tolerability profile of zolmitriptan (Zomig; 311C90), a novel dual central and peripherally acting 5HT1B/1D agonist. Cephalalgia 17: 41–52
64. Rolan P (1997) Potential drug interactions with the novel antimigraine compound zolmitriptan (Zomig (R), 311C90). Cephalalgia 17[Suppl 18]: 21–27
65. Peck RW, Seaber EJ, Dixon R, Gillotin CG, Weatherley BC, Layton G, Posner J (1997) The interaction between propranolol and the novel antimigraine agent zolmitriptan (311C90). Br J Clin Pharmacol 44: 595–599
66. Cutler NR, Claghorn J, Sramek JJ, Block G, Panebianco D, Cheng H, Olah TV, Reines SA (1996) Pilot study of MK-462 in migraine. Cephalalgia 16: 113–116
67. Visser WH, Terwindt GM, Reines SA, Jiang K, Lines CR, Ferrari MD, for the Dutch/U.S. Rizatriptan Study Group (1997) Rizatriptan vs sumatriptan in the acute treatment of migraine. A placebo-controlled, dose-ranging study. Arch Neurol 53: 1132–1137
68. Teall J, Tuchmann M, Cutler N, Gross M, Willoughby E, Smith B, Jiang K, Reines S, Block G, on behalf of the Rizatriptan 022 Study Group (1998) Rizatriptan (MAXALT) for the acute treatment of migraine and migraine recurrence. A placebo-controlled, outpatient study. Headache 38: 281–287
69. Tfelt-Hansen P, Teall J, Rodriguez F, Giacovazzo M, Paz J, Malbecq W, Block GA, Reines SA, Visser WH, on behalf of the Rizatriptan 030 Study Group (1998) Oral rizatriptan versus oral sumatriptan: a direct comparative study in the acute treatment of migraine. Headache 38: 748–755
70. Goldstein J, Ryan R, Jiang K, Getson A, Norman B, Block G, Lines C, and the Rizatriptan Protocol 046 Study Group (1998) Crossover comparison of rizatriptan 5 mg and 10 mg versus sumatriptan 25 and 50 mg in migraine. Headache 38: 737–747
71. Kramer MS, Matzura-Wolfe D, Polis A, Getson A, Amaraneni PG, Solbach MP, McHugh W, Feighner J, Silberstein S, Reines SA, and the Rizatriptan Multiple Attack Study Group (1998) A placebo-controlled crossover study of rizatriptan in the treatment of multiple migraine attacks. Neurology 51: 773–781
72. Pascual J, Vega P, Diener HC, Allen C, Vrijens F, Patel K, and the Rizatriptan-Zolmitriptan Study Group (2000) Comparison of rizatriptan 10 mg vs. zolmitriptan 2.5 mg in the acute treatment of migraine. Cephalalgia 20: 455–461
73. Bomhof M, Paz J, Legg N, Allen C, Vandormael K, Patel K (1999) Comparison of rizatriptan 10 mg vs. naratriptan 2.5 mg in migraine. Eur Neurol 42: 173–179
74. Goadsby PJ (2000) Rizatriptan in acute treatment of migraine: update on new comparative data. Cephalalgia 20[Suppl 1]: 10–15
75. Ahrens SP, Farmer MV, Williams DL, Willoughby E, Jiang K, Block GA, Visser WH, and the Rizatriptan Wafer Protocol 049 Study Group (1999) Efficacy and

safety of rizatriptan wafer for the acute treatment of migraine. Cephalalgia 19: 525–530
76. Adelman JU, Mannix LK, Seggern von RL (2000) Rizatriptan tablet versus wafer: patient preference. Headache 40: 371–372
77. Klapper JA, O'Connor S (2000) Rizatriptan wafer-sublingual vs. placebo at the onset of acute migraine. Cephalalgia 20: 585–587
78. Diener HC, McHarg A (2000) Pharmacology and efficacy of eletriptan for the treatment of migraine attacks. Int J Clin Pract 54: 670–674
79. Färkkilä M, Diener HC, Dahlöf C, Steiner TJ, on behalf of the Eletriptan Steering Committee (1996) A dose-finding study of eletriptan (5–30 mg) for the acute treatment of migraine. Cephalalgia 16: 387
80. Goadsby PJ, Ferrari MD, Olesen J, Stovner LJ, Senard JM, Jackson NC, Poole PH, for the Eletriptan Steering Committee (2000) Eletriptan in acute migraine: a double-blind, placebo-controlled comparison to sumatriptan. Neurology 54: 156–163
81. Steiner TJ, on behalf of the Eletriptan Steering Committee (1998) The efficacy, saftey and tolerability of oral eletriptan (40 mg and 80 mg) for the acute treatment of migraine: results of a double-blind, placebo-controlled, parallel group clinical trial. Migraine Trust, London
82. Diener HC, Reches A, Pascual J, Jansen J-P, Pitei D, Steiner T, on behalf of the Eletriptan and Cafergot Comparative Study Group (2002) Efficacy, tolerability and safety of oral eletriptan and ergotamine plus caffeine (Cafergot) in the acute treatment of migraine: a multicentre, randomised, double-blind, placebo-controlled comparison. Eur Neurol 47: 99–107
83. Cabarrocas X, Zayas JM, on behalf of the Almotriptan Oral Study Group (1998) Efficacy data on oral almotriptan, a novel 5-HT1B/D agonist. Headache 38: 377
84. Pascual J (2000) Therapy with other triptans: almotriptan. In: Diener HC (ed) Drug treatment of migraine and other headaches. Karger, Basel, pp 197–205
85. Pascual J, Falk RM, Piessens F, Prusinski A, Docekal P, Robert M, Ferrer P, Luria X, Segarra R, Zayas JM (2000) Consistent efficacy and tolerability of almotriptan in the acute treatment of multiple migraine attacks: results of a large, randomized, double-blind, placebo-controlled study. Cephalalgia 20: 588–596
86. Cabarrocas X, Zayas JM, Suris M, on behalf of the Almotriptan Oral Study Group (1998) Equivalent efficacy of oral almotriptan, a new 5-HT1B/D agonist, compared with sumatriptan 100 mg. Headache 38: 377–378
87. Spierings E, Gomez-Mancilla B, Grosz D, Rowland C, Whaley F, Jirgens K (2001) Oral almotriptan vs. oral sumatriptan in the abortive treatment of migraine: a double-blind, randomized, parallel-group, optimum-dose comparison. Arch Neurol 58: 944–950
88. Mathew NT, for the Oral Almotriptan Study Group (2002) A long-term open-label study of oral almotriptan 12.5 mg for the treatment of acute migraine. Headache 42: 32–40
89. Cabarrocas X, Esbri R, Peris F, Ferrer P (2001) Long-term efficacy and safety of oral almotriptan: interim analysis of a 1-year open study. Headache 41: 57–62
90. Brown AM, Ho M, Thomas DR, Parson AA (1998) Comparison of functional effects of frovatriptan, sumatriptan and naratriptan on human recombinant 5-HT1 and 5-HT7 receptors. Headache 38: 376
91. Goldstein J, Elkind A, Keywood C, Klapper J, Ryan R (1998) A low dose range-finding study of frovatriptan: a potent selective 5-HT1B/D agonist for the acute treatment of migraine. Headache 38: 382–383
92. Goldstein J, Keywood C, 251/96/14 Study Group (2002) Frovatriptan for the acute treatment of migraine: a dose-finding study. Headache 42: 41–48
93. The International Headache Society Committee on Clinical Trials in Migraine (1991) Guidelines for controlled trials of drugs in migraine 1st edn. Cephalalgia 11: 1–12

94. Pilgrim AJ (1991) Methodology of clinical trials of sumatriptan in migraine and cluster headache. Eur Neurol 31: 295–299
95. Tfelt-Hansen P (1998) Efficacy and adverse events of subcutaneous, oral, and intranasal sumatriptan used for migraine treatment: a systematic review based on number needed to treat. Cephalalgia 18: 532–538
96. Ferrari MD (1999) The war of the triptans. Teaching course, Syllabus, EFNS, Lisbon
97. Stark S, Spierings ELH, McNiel S, Putnam GP, Bolden-Watson CP, O'Quinn S (2000) Naratriptan efficacy in migraineurs who respond poorly to oral sumatriptan. Headache 40: 513–520
98. Visser WH, Jaspers N, de Vriend RHM, Ferrari MD (1996) Risk factors for headache recurrence after sumatriptan: a study in 366 migraine patients. Cephalalgia 16: 264–269
99. McDavis HL, Hutchison J, Frovatriptan Phase III Investigators (1999) Frovatriptan — a review of overall clinical efficacy. Cephalalgia 19: 363–364
100. Diener HC, Tfelt-Hansen P (1993) Headache associated with chronic use of substances. In: Olesen J, Tfelt-Hansen P, Welch KMA (eds) The headaches. Raven Press, New York, pp 721–727
101. Kaube H, May A, Diener HC, Pfaffenrath V (1994) Sumatriptan misuse in daily chronic headache. BMJ 308: 1573
102. Gaist D, Hallas J, Sindrup SH, Gram LF (1996) Is overuse of sumatriptan a problem? A population-based study. Eur J Clin Pharmacol 3: 161–165
103. Gaist D, Tsiropoulus I, Sindrup SH, Hallas J, Rasmussen BK, Kragstrup J (1998) Inappropriate use of sumatriptan: population based register and interview study. Br J Med 316: 1352–1353
104. Gaist D (1999) Use and overuse of sumatriptan. Pharmaco-epidemiological studies based on prescription register and interview data. Cephalalgia 19: 735–761
105. Katsarava Z, Fritsche G, Diener HC, Limmroth V (2000) Drug-induced headache (DIH) following the use of different triptans. Cephalalgia 20: 293 [abstract]
106. Limmroth V, Kazarawa S, Fritsche G, Diener HC (1999) Headache after frequent use of new 5-HT agonists zolmitriptan and naratriptan. Lancet 353: 378
107. MaassenVanDenBrink A, Reekers M, Bax WA, Ferrari MD, Saxena PR (1998) Coronary side-effect potential of current and prospective antimigraine drugs. Circulation 98: 25–30
108. MassenVanDenBrink A, Bax WA, Ramrattan NN, Ferrari MD, Saxena PR (1999). Human isolated coronary artery contraction to sumatriptan: a post hoc analysis. Cephalagia 19: 651–654
109. Cady RK, Lipton RB, Hall C, Stewart WF, O'Quinn S, Gutterman D (2001) Treatment of mild headache in disabled migraine sufferers: results of the Spectrum study. Headache 40: 792–797
110. Diener HC, for the RPR100893-201 Migraine Study Group (1995) Substance P antagonist RPR100893-201 is not effective in human migraine attacks. 6th International Headache Research Seminar, Copenhagen, pp 245–371
111. Goldstein DJ, Wang O, Saper JR, Stoltz R, Silberstein ST, Mathew NT (1997) Ineffectiveness of neurokinin-1 antagonist in acute migraine: crossover study. Cephalalgia 17: 785–790
112. May A, Gijsman HJ, Wallnöfer A, Jones R, Diener HC, Ferrari MD (1996) Endothelin antagonist bosentan blocks neurogenic inflammation, but is not effective in aborting migraine attacks. Pain 67: 375–378
113. Lassen LH, Ashina M, Christiansen I, Ulrich V, Grover R, Donaldson J, Olesen J (1998) Nitric oxide synthase inhibition: a new principle in the treatment of migraine attacks. Cephalalgia 18: 27–32
114. Ramadan N, Sang C, Chappell A, Vandenhende F, Johnson K, Phebus L, Bleakman D, Ornstein P, Arnold B, Freitag F, Smith T, Silberstein S, Tepper S (2001) IV LY293558, an AMPA/KA receptor antagonist, is effective in migraine. Cephalalgia 21: 267

115. Phebus LA, Johnson KW, Zgombick JL, et al. (1997) Characterization of LY334370 as a pharmacological tool to study 5HT1F receptors binding affinities, brain penetration and activity in the neurogenic dural inflammation model of migraine. Life Sci 61: 2117–2126
116. Goldstein DJ, Roon KI, Offen WW, Ramadan NM, Phebus LA, Johnson KW, Schaus JM, Ferrari MD (2001) Selective serotonine 1F ($5\text{-}HT_{1F}$) receptor agonist LY334370 for acute migraine: a randomised controlled trial. Lancet 358: 1230–1234
117. Lipton RB, Stewart WF, Ryan RE, Saper J, Silberstein S, Sheftell F (1998) Efficacy and safety of acetaminophen, aspirin, and caffeine in alleviating migraine headache pain — Three double-blind, randomized, placebo-controlled trials. Arch Neurol 55: 210–217
118. Myllylä VV, Havanka H, Herrala L, Kangasniemi P, Rautakorpi I, Turkka J, Vapaatalo H, Eskerod O (1998) Tolfenamic acid rapid release versus sumatriptan in the acute treatment of migraine: comparable effect in a double-blind, randomized, controlled, prallel-group study. Headache 38: 201–207
119. Tfelt-Hansen P, Henry P, Mulder LJ, Schaeldewaert RG, Schoenen J, Chazot G (1995) The effectiveness of combined oral lysine acetylsalicylate and metoclopramide compared with oral sumatriptan for migraine. Lancet 346: 923–926
120. Codispoti JR, Prior MJ, Fu M, Harte CM, Nelson EB (2001) Efficacy of nonprescription doses of ibuprofen for treating migraine headache. A randomized controlled trial. Headache 41: 665–679
121. Dahlöf C, Björkman R (1993) Diclofenac-K (50 and 100 mg) and placebo in the acute treatment of migraine. Cephalalgia 13: 117–123
122. Karachalios GN, Fotiadou A, Chrisikos N, Karabetsos A, Kehagioglou K (1992) Treatment of acute migraine attack with diclofenac sodium: a double-blind study. Headache 32: 98–100
123. The Diclofenac-K/Sumatriptan Migraine Study Group (1999) Acute treatment of migraine attacks: efficacy and safety of a nonsteroidal antiinflammatory drug, diclofenac-potassium, in comparison to oral sumatriptan and placebo. Cephalalgia 19: 232–240
124. de Craen AJM, Tijssen JGP, de Gans J, Kleijnen J (2000) Placebo effect in the acute treatment of migraine: subcutaneous placebos are better than oral placebos. J Neurol 247: 183–188
125. McQuay H, Carroll D, Moore A (1995) Variation in the placebo effect in randomised controlled trials of analgesics: all is as blind as it seems. Pain 64: 331–335
126. Migraine-Nimodipine European Study Group M (1989) European multicenter trial of nimodipine in the prophylaxis of common migraine (migraine without aura). Headache 29: 633–638
127. Migraine-Nimodipine European Study Group M (1989) European multicenter trial of nimodipine in the prophylaxis of classic migraine (migraine with aura). Headache 29: 639–642
128. Couch JR (1987) Placebo effect and clinical trials in migraine therapy. Neuroepidemiology 6: 178–185
129. Rabkin R, Stables DP, Levin NW, Suzman MM (1966) The prophylactic value of propranolol in angina pectoris. Am J Cardiol 18: 370–383
130. Holroyd KA, Penzien DB, Cordingley GE (1991) Propranolol in the management of recurrent migraine: a meta-analytic review. Headache 31: 333–340
131. Kangasniemi P, Hedman C (1984) Metoprolol and propranolol in the prophylactic treatment of classical and common migraine. A double-blind study. Cephalalgia 4: 91–96
132. Ljung O (1980) Treatment of migraine with metoprolol. N Engl J Med 303(3): 664–668
133. Steiner TJ, Joseph R, Hedman C, Clifford Rose F (1988) Metoprolol in the prophylaxis of migraine: parallel group comparison with placebo and dose-ranging follow-up. Headache 28: 15–23

134. Olsson JE, Behring HC, Forssman B, Hedman C, Hedman G, Johansson F, Kinnman J, Palhagen SE, Samuelsson M, Strandman E (1984) Metoprolol and propranolol in migraine prophylaxis: a double-blind multicenter study. Acta Neurol Scand 70: 160–168
135. Sorensen PS, and the Danish Migraine Study Group (1989) Prophylactic effect of flunarizine versus metoprolol in migraine. Cephalalgia 9: 355–356
136. Sorensen PS, Larsen BH, Rasmussen MJK, Kinge E, Iversen H, Alslev T, Nohr P, Pedersen KK, Schroder P, Lademann A, Olesen J (1991) Flunarizine versus metoprolol in migraine prophylaxis: a double-blind, randomized parallel group study of efficacy and tolerability. Headache 31: 650–657
137. Vilming S, Standnes B, Hedman C (1985) Metoprolol and pizotifen in the prophylactic treatment of classical and common migraine. A double-blind investigation. Cephalalgia 5: 17–23
138. Wörz R, Reinhardt-Benmalek B, Grotemeyer KH, Foh M (1991) Bisoprolol and metoprolol in the prophylactic treatment of migraine with and without aura — a randomized double-blind cross-over multicenter study. Cephalalgia 11[Suppl 11]: 152–153
139. Gawel MJ, Kreeft J, Nelson RF, Simard D, Arnott WS (1992) Comparison of the efficacy and safety of flunarizine to propranolol in the prophylaxis of migraine. Can J Neurol Sci 19: 340–345
140. Holroyd KA, Penzien DB, Rokicki LA, Cordingley GE (1992) Flunarizine vs propranolol: a meta-analysis of clinical trials. Headache 32: 256
141. Ludin H-P (1989) Flunarizine and propranolol in the treatment of migraine. Headache 29: 218–223
142. Lücking CH, Oestreich W, Schmidt R, Soyka D (1988) Flunarizine vs. propranolol in the prophylaxis of migraine: two double-blind comparative studies in more than 400 patients. Cephalalgia 8: 21–26
143. Shimell CJ, Fritz VU, Levien SL (1990) A comparative trial of flunarizine and propranolol in the prevention of migraine. S Afr Med J 77: 75–78
144. Forssman B, Lindblad CJ, Zbornikova V (1983) Atenolol for migraine prophylaxis. Headache 23: 188–190
145. Stensrud P, Sjaastad O (1980) Comparative trial of Tenormin (atenolol) and Inderal (propranolol) in migraine. Headache 20: 204–207
146. Briggs RS, Millac PA (1979) Timolol in migraine prophylaxis. Headache 19: 379–381
147. Stellar S, Ahrens S, Meibohm AR, Reines AS (1984) Migraine prevention with timolol. A double-blind crossover study. Jama 252: 2576–2580
148. Tfelt-Hansen P, Standnes B, Kangasniemi P, Hakkarainen H, Olesen J (1984) Timolol vs. propranolol vs. placebo in common migraine prophylaxis: a double-blind multicenter trial. Acta Neurol Scand 69: 1–8
149. Freitag FG, Diamond S (1984) Nadolol and placebo comparison study in the prophylactic treatment of migraine. J Am Osteopath Assoc 84: 343–347
150. van de Ven LLM, Franke CL, Koehler PJ, on Behalf of the Investigators (1997) Prophylactic treatment of migraine with bisoprolol: a placebo-controlled study. Cephalalgia 17: 596–599
151. Wörz R, Reinhard-Benmalek B, Foeh M, Grotemeyer KH, Scharafinski HW (1992) Migraine prophylaxis with bisoprolol. Headache Quarterly 3: 64–72
152. Olesen J, Tfelt-Hansen P, Welch KMA (eds) (1998) The headaches, 2nd ed. Raven Press, New York
153. Diener HC (2000) Flunarizine for migraine prophylaxis. In: Diener HC (ed) Drug treatment of migraine and other headaches. Karger, Basel, pp 269–278
154. Markley HG, Cheronis CD, Piepho RW (1984) Verapamil in prophylactic therapy of migraine. Neurology 34: 973–976
155. Solomon CGD, Steel MJG, Spaccavento CLJ (1983) Verapamil prophylaxis of migraine. Jama 250: 2500–2502

156. Scholz E, Gerber WD, Diener HC, Langohr HD, Reinecke M (1987) Dihydroergotamine versus flunarizine versus nifedipine versus metoprolol versus propranolol in migraine prophylaxis. A comparative study based on time series analysis. In: Clifford Rose F (ed) Advances in headache research. John Libbey & Co, London, pp 135–145
157. Albers GW, Simon LT, Hamik A, Peroutka SJ (1989) Nifedipine versus propranolol for the initial prophylaxis of migraine. Headache 29: 214–217
158. Diener H, Krupp P, Schmitt T, Steitz G, Milde K, Freytag S, on behalf of the Study Group (2001) Cyclandelate in the prophylaxis of migraine: a placebo-controlled study. Cephalalgia 21: 66–70
159. Neumann M, Demarez JP, Harmey JL, Le Bastard B, Cauquil J (1986) Prevention of migraine attacks through the use of dihydroergotamine. Int J Clin Pharm Res 6: 11–13
160. Grotemeyer K-H, Schlake H-P, Husstedt IW (1989) Etilefrine pivalate vs. dihydroergotamin and flunarizin in prophylactic treatment of migraine in patients with low blood pressure — a randomized double-blind-study. Cephalalgia 9: 433–434
161. Silberstein SD (1998) Methysergide. Cephalalgia 18: 421–435
162. Buring JE, Peto R, Hennekens CH (1990) Low-dose aspirin for migraine prophylaxis. JAMA 264: 1711–1713
163. Grotemeyer K, Scharafinski H, Schlake H, Husstedt IW (1990) Acetylsalicylic acid vs metoprolol in migraine prophylaxis — a double blind cross-over study. Headache 30: 639–641
164. Diener HC, Hartung E, Chrubasik J, Evers S, Schoenen J, Gendolla AGL, Hauke W, for the Study Group (2001) A comparative study of acetylsalicyclic acid and metoprolol for the prophylactic treatment of migraine. A randomised, controlled, double-blind, parallel group phase III study. Cephalalgia 21: 140–144
165. Bensenor IM, Cook NR, Lee I-M, Chown MJ, Hennekens CH, Buring JE (2001) Low-dose aspirin for migraine prophylaxis in women. Cephalalgia 21: 175–183
166. Ziegler DK, Ellis DJ (1985) Naproxen in prophylaxis of migraine. Arch Neurol 42: 582–584
167. Behan PO, Connelly K (1986) Prophylaxis of migraine: a comparison between naproxen sodium and pizotifen. Headache 26: 237–239
168. Bellavance AJ, Meloche JP (1990) Comparative study of naproxen sodium, pizotyline and placebo in migraine prophylaxis. Headache 30: 710–715
169. Sargent J, Solbach P, Damasio H, Baumel B, Corbett J, Eisner L, Jessen B, Kudrow L, Mathew N, Medina J, Saper J, Vijayan N, Watson C, Alger J (1985) A comparison of naproxen sodium to propranolol hydrochloride and a placebo control for the prophylaxis of migraine headache. Headache 25: 320–324
170. Sances G, Martignoni E, Fioroni L, Blandini F, Facchinetti F, Nappi G (1990) Naproxen sodium in menstrual migraine prophylaxis: a double-blind placebo controlled study. Headache 30: 705–709
171. Diamond S, Freitag FG, Gallagher RM, Feinberg DT (1990) Ketoprofen in the prophylaxis of migraine. Headache Quarterly 1: 75–77
172. Johnson RH, Hornabrook RW, Lambie DG (1986) Comparison of mefenamic acid and propranolol with placebo in migraine prophylaxis. Acta Neurol Scand 73: 490–492
173. Mikkelsen B, Pedersen KK, Christiansen LV (1986) Prophylactic treatment of migraine with tolfenamic acid, propranolol and placebo. Acta Neurol Scand 73: 423–427
174. Couch JR, Hassanein RS (1979) Amitriptyline in migraine prophylaxis. Arch Neurol 36: 695–699
175. Ziegler DK, Hurwitz A, Hassanein RS (1987) Migraine prophylaxis. A comparison of propranolol and amitriptyline. Arch Neurol 44: 486–489

176. Ziegler DK, Hurwitz A, Preskorn S, Hassanein R, Seim J (1993) Propranolol and amitriptyline in prophylaxis of migraine. Arch Neurol 50: 825–830
177. Bussone G, Cerbo R, Martucci N, Micieli G, Zanferrari C, Grazzi L, Fabbrini G, Cavallini A, Granella F, Ambrosoli L, Mailland F, Poli A, Manzoni G (1999) Alpha-dihydroergocryptine in the prophylaxis of migraine: a multicenter double-blind study versus flunarizine. Headache 39: 426–431
178. Peikert A, Wilimzig C, Köhne-Volland R (1996) Prophylaxis of migraine with oral magnesium: results from a prospective, multi-center, placebo-controlled and double-blind randomized study. Cephalalgia 16: 257–263
179. Pfaffenrath V, Wessely P, Meyer C, Isler HR, Evers S, Grotemeyer KH, Taneri Z, Soyka D, Göbel H, Fischer M (1996) Magnesium in the prophylaxis of migraine — a double-blind, placebo-controlled study. Cephalalgia 16: 436–440
180. Schoenen J, Lenaerts M, Bastings E (1994) High-dose riboflavin as a prophylactic treatment of migraine: results of an open pilot study. Cephalalgia 14: 328–330
181. Schoenen J, Jacquy J, Lenaerts M (1997) High-dose power riboflavin as a novel prophylactic antimigraine therapy: results from a double-blind, randomized, placebo-controlled trial. Cephalalgia 17: 244
182. Silberstein S, Mathew N, Saper J, Jenkins S, for the BOTOX Migraine Clinical Research Group (2000) Botulinum toxin type A as a migraine preventive treatment. Headache 40: 445–450
183. Hering R, Kurzitzky A (1992) Sodium valproate in the prophylactic treatment of migraine: a double-blind study versus placebo. Cephalalgia 12: 81–84
184. Jensen R, Brinck T, Olesen J (1994) Sodium valproate has a prophylactic effect in migraine without aura: a triple-blind, placebo-controlled crossover study. Neurology 44: 647–651
185. Kaniecki RG (1997) A comparision of divalproex with propranolol and placebo for the prophylaxis of migraine without aura. Arch Neurol 54: 1141–1145
186. Klapper J, on behalf of the Divalproex Sodium in Migraine Prophylaxis Study Group (1997) Divalproex sodium in migraine prophylaxis: a dose-controlled study. Cephalalgia 17: 103–108
187. Mathew NT, Saper JR, Silberstein SD, Rankin L, Markley HG, Solomon S, Rapoport AM, Silber CJ, Deaton RL (1995) Migraine prophylaxis with divalproex. Arch Neurol 52: 281–286
188. Steiner TJ, Findley LJ, Yuen AWC (1997) Lamotrigine versus placebo in the prophylaxis of migraine with and without aura. Cephalalgia 17: 109–112
189. Lampl C, Buzath A, Klinger D, Neumann K (1999) Lamotrigine in the prophylactic treatment of migraine aura — a pilot study. Cephalalgia 19: 58–63
190. Mathew NT, Rapoport A, Saper J, Magnus L, Klapper J, Ramadan N, Stacey B, Tepper S (2001) Efficacy of gabapentin in migraine prophylaxis. Headache 41: 119–128
191. Potter DL, Hart DE, Calder CS, Storey JR (2000) A double-blind, randomized, placebo-controlled, parallel study to determine the efficacy of topiramate in the prophylactic treatment of migraine. Neurology 54[Suppl 3]: A15
192. Shuaib A, Ahmed F, Muratoglu M, Kochanski P (1999) Topiramate in migraine prophylaxis: a pilot study. Cephalalgia 19(4): 379–380
193. Shuaib A (2000) Efficacy of topiramate in prophylaxis of frequent severe migraines or chornic daily headaches: experience with 68 patients over 18 months. Cephalalgia 20: 423
194. Storey JR, Calder CS, Hart DE, Potter DL (2001) Topiramate in migraine prevention: a double-blind, placebo-controlled study. Headache 41: 968–975
195. Newman LC, Lipton RB, Lay CL, Solomon S (1998) A pilot study of oral sumatriptan as intermittent prophylaxis of menstruation-related migraine. Neurology 51: 307–309
196. Newman L, Mannix LK, Landy S, Silberstein S, Lipton RB, Pait Putnam DG, Watson C, Jöbsis M, Batenhorst A, O'Quinn S (2001) Naratriptan as short-term

prophylaxis in menstrually associated migraine: a randomised, double-blind, placebo-controlled study. Headache 41: 248–256
197. Pradalier A, Vincent D, Beaulieu PH, Baudesson G, Launay JM (1994) Correlation between between oestradiol plasma level and therapeutic effect on menstrual migraine. In: Clifford-Rose F (ed) New advances in headache research. Smith-Gordon, London, pp 129–132
198. Hershey AD, Powers SW, Bentti AL, Grauw de TJ (2000) Effectiveness of amitriptyline in the prophylactic management of childhood headaches. Headache 40: 539–549
199. Lanzi G, Balottin U, Zambrino CA, Cernibori A, Del Bene E, Gallai V, Guidetti V, Sorge F (1996) Guidelines and recommendations for the treatment of migraine in pediatric and adolescent patients. Funct Neurol 11: 269–275

Author's address: Prof. Dr. H.-Ch. Diener, Department of Neurology, University Essen, Hufelandstrasse 55, D-45122 Essen, Federal Republic of Germany, e-mail: h.diener@uni-essen.de

J Neural Transm (2003) [Suppl] 64: 65–78

Advances in the pharmacological management of Parkinson disease

E. Tolosa

Neurology Service, ICMSN, and Banco de Tejidos Neurológicos, Hospital Clinico, University of Barcelona, Barcelona, Spain

Summary. Numerous advances have taken place in the pharmacological management of Parkinson disease (PD) in recent years. Some of the more clinically relevant will be discussed in the text that follows. New drugs have been developed to treat or prevent the motor fluctuations and dyskinesias that occur frequently with the continuous use of levodopa. Such drugs include the catechol-O-methyl-transferase (COMT) inhibitors, such as tolcapone and entecapone, and new dopamine (DA) agonists with long half lives such as cabergoline, pramipexole or ropirinole. Also new, atyical, antipsychotics have appeared which have revolutionized the treatment of PD since they allow us to control hallucinations and other psychotic behaviour without worsening of motor function. Finally preliminary reports suggest that cholinesterase inhibitors, such as rivastigmine, can be usefull in the management of cognitive impairment in PD, one of the most difficult clinical problems encountered in the management of this neurodegenerative disorder.

Introduction

Levodopa, a precursor of DA, has been the most effective symptomatic treatment of PD for the las three decades (Cotzias et al., 1970; Papavasiliou et al., 1972; Tolosa, 1998). Levodopa is coadministered with a peripheral amino acid decarboxylase inhibitor (carbidopa or benserazide) to improve its peripheral pharmacokinetics and to reduce the adverse events associated with increase peripheral DA. It improves all patients with PD and improves all symptoms including tremor and gait and equilibrium dysfunction (Agid et al., 1999).

Drawbacks of levodopa treatment include dyskinesias, fluctuations in motor performance such as wearing off and on-off, and psychiatric side effects such as hallucinations, intermittent confusion or paranoia (Tolosa et al., 1975; Fahn, 1974; Marsden et al., 1982; Nutt, 1990). These complications arise in approximatley 25 to 50% of patients after approximately 5 years of long term treatment. Motor complications are more prevalent in young onset patients. Dyskinesias, once developed tend to persist or recurr promptly if treatment is restarted later even if it had been discontinued for months ("priming" effect). Psychiatric side effects occur more frequently in the elderly and in the more advanced stages of the illness.

The limitations encountered during levodopa treatment have led over the years to the development of new formulations of levodopa and of newer antiparkinsoninan agents such monoamine-oxidase type B inhibitors, COMT inhibitors and DA agonists (Tolosa et al., 1994). They also have prompted debates about whether or not the initiation of treatment with levodopa should be delayed. Some of these new drugs and issues will be discussed in the text that follows.

COMT inhibitors in the treatment of Parkinson disease

After oral administration levodopa is metabolized in the periphery through decarboxylation. Less than 1% of an oral dose eventually reaches the brain. O-methylation is the second most important metabolic pathway. Approximately 10% of levodopa is converted to 3-O methyldopa (Nutt and Fellman, 1984). Combining levodopa with a dopa decarboxylase inhibitor such as carbidopa or benserazide increases plasma levodopa levels to 14 times the peak levels and the amount of levodopa entering the brain is increased by 5 to 10%. With decarboxylase inhibition metablism of levodopa is shifted largely towards COMT which is widely distributed in tissues including brain, gut, kidney, liver and erythrocites (Kuruma et al., 1971). Therefore, peripheral COMT inhibition should increase the bioavailability of levodopa and increase its half-life (Männistö and Kaakkola, 1989; Männistö et al., 1992; Goetz, 1998; Kurth and Adler, 1998). Several studies have shown that COMT inhibitors improve the pharmacokinetics of levodopa increasing its bioavilability. The maximum plasma concentration (Cmax) is, however, not changed which suggest that levodopa will last longer, be more available to the brain but not have a higher incidence of peak-dose side effects. Centrally active COMT inhibitors, such as tolcapone, could also extend the beneficial effect of levodopa by blocking the metabolic degradation of dopamine in the striatum in a way similar to the results obtained with the use of a MAO-B inhibitor (Männistö, 1994).

Two double blind placebo controlled studies co-administering tolcapone to levodopa three times a day have shown increased "on" time of about 25%, decreased "off" time of 32 to 48% and reductions of daily levodopa dose of arround 20%. No tolerance to the beneficial effects of this drug have occured in trials lasting up to one year. Parkinson disease patients with a stable response to levodopa also improve on tolcapone, but additional trials are needed to confirm that stable responders to levodopa benefit on the long run of the coadministration of a COMT inhibitor (Rajput et al., 1997; Adler et al., 1998). Tolcapone elimination half-life is 2 hours and dosing is needed only three times a day.

Entecapone is a peripherally acting selective, reversible COMT inhibitor. Both open-labled and double-blind trials have shown the effectiveness of entecapone. This peripheral inhibitor increased the plasma concentration vs time curve of levodopa by 35% and increased the half life by 32% but did not alter the maximum concentration of levodopa compared with placebo. Entecapone incresed the duration of "on" time in response to a single dose of levodopa by 24% and increased the total daily "on" time based on patients diary evaluations by 23% compared with placebo. Entecapone is a short acting drug and must be given with each dose of levodopa (Keränen et al., 1996; Rinne et al., 1998; Parkinson Study Group, 1997).

The most common adverse effects of COMT inhibitors are related to their ability to potentiate the effects of levodopa. In all studies the most commonly seen dopaminergic adverse effect was a worsening of levodopa — induced dyskinesias. This may be minimized in most patients by a downward adjustment of the levodopa dosage. Orthostatic hypotention, nausea and vomiting and psychosis may also be seen.

Tolcapone has been associated with diarrhea in approx 17% of cases. It may be severe and require discontinuation of the drug. The mechanism of this adverse effect is not yet understood but it does not appear to be dose dependent. Entecapone rarely causes diarrhoea but can cause constipation. Both entecapone and tolcapone frequently cause a benign discoloration of the urine that may alarm patients unless they are informed of this potential effect prior to treatment.

Tolcapone has rarely been associated with transient elevation of transaminase levels. With its use, though, several cases of fatal hepatotoxicity ocurred and the drug has been temporarily suspended in most countries. Entecapone does not seem to suffer from this problem.

In summary, although the COMT inhibitors reduce the total daily administered dose of levodopa they should not be considered levodopa sparing drugs since they increase the plasma concentration — time curve of levodopa. Since these drugs increase the plasma availability of levodopa without increasing its maximum concentration there appears to be a definite advantage over just raising the dosage of levodopa administered. The introduction in the clinic of well tolerated COMT inhibitors is a significant development for those treating advanced PD patients suffering from levodopa-induced motor fluctuations and possibly for stable patients as well. These drugs have been used in conjunction with the DA agonists and selegiline and it is very likely that their role will be as an adjunct to these drugs combined to levodopa. Currently only entecapone is available to treat PD patients since tolcapone was suspended due to liver toxicity.

Expanding role of the dopamine agonists

The appearance of motor fluctuations and dyskinesias in patients treated with levodopa promted the introduction of DA agonists as an adjunct treatment to levodopa in patients with advanced PD. Numerous studies have shown that direct acting agonists that stimulate DA D2 receptors are an excellent adjuvant treatment to levodopa in patients who develop these motor alterations

(Tolosa and Marin, 1997). In most patients introduction of an agonist results in longer "on" period, less severe "off"'s, and generally less dyskinesias, particularly early morning dystonia. Night time mobility also frequently improves. DA agonist treatment frequently requires decreasing the dose of levodopa although in some patients this is not required. In other patients, on the contrary, with extreme sensitivity to DA, the dose of levodopa is reduced to a bare minimum (Sànchez-Ramos, 1997). The major drawbacks of DA agonists are the increased incidence of hallucinations and delusions and rarely postural hypotension and erythromelalgia. Nausea is common at the initiation of treatment but with the use of domperidone can usually be averted. Side effects of the DA agonists are dose-dependent and reversible (Tolosa and Marin, 1997; Tolosa, 1999).

More recently DA agonists are being introduced earlier in the management plan since their use is rarely associated to dyskinesias and fluctuations and have proved effective in the early stages as monotherapy in patients with mild symptoms. Introducing DA agonists in the initial stages of the illness may allow delaying the introduction of levodopa for several months, forestalling the development of motor complications. Such early use of an agonist is considered advantageous also in other ways. For those who suscribe to the oxidative stress theory of cell death in PD, for example, DA agonists would reduce the turnover of DA in remaining nigral neurons and would not be associated with further increase in oxidative metabolism of DA encouraged by the use of levodopa. Preclinical studies suggest, furthermore, that some of the new agonists could indeed have a neuroprotective effect.

DA agonists in early Parkinson disease

The benefit of the agonists as monotherapy in mild PD has been shown in large, prospective, double — blind, placebo controlled trials. In these trials ropinirole, pramipexole, cabergoline or pergolide, used as monotherapy provided antiparkinsonian benefits to early PD superior to placebo. These benefits are particularly powerfull in patients with Hoehn and Yahr stages I and II and, in some studies, comparable to levodopa (Tolosa et al., 1987; Rascol et al., 1982; Adler et al., 1997; Sethi et al., 1998; Kieburtz et al., 1997; Shannon et al., 1997; Rinne et al., 1997).

Subsequently single monotherapy trials (large, multicentric prospective double blind) comparing these agonists against levodopa have been performed (Rascol et al., 2000; Parkinson Study Group, 2000; Rinne et al., 1998). In each of these studies patients randomized to initiate therapy with the DA agonist had significantly fewer motor complications than patients treated with levodopa alone. Patients randomized to the agonist arm though, had less improvement in motor impairments and or disability. These differences may reflect the fact that levodopa is the most effective antiparkinsonian agent but it is also possible that dopamine agonists provided benefits that are not captured by the UPDRS scales. In terms of tolerability hallucinations were significantly worse with ropinirole and somnolence with pramipexole.

Withdrawals because of adverse events were greater with the agonists than with levodopa.

As similar results have been obtained with each of the DA agonists studied, it is likely that this benefit is a class effect that can be seen with all long acting DA receptor agonists. These studies support a treatment strategy for early PD in which DA agonists are used as initial therapy and supplemental levodopa is added when symptoms cannot be satisfactorily controlled with a DA agonist as monotherapy.

In summary DA agonists have been used since their introduction into the therapy of PD as adjuvants to levodopa in patients with motor fluctuations and dyskinesias. Based on accumulating preclinical and clinical evidence suggesting that its use offers advantages over levodopa in the treatment of early PD they are now frequently used in the early management of this disease. Recent, well conducted studies with the new generation of DA agonists have shown that the agonists are effective in controling motor disability as monotherapy in early stages when disease severity is mild. Most neurologists would initiate treatment of a young patient, prone to develop early and severe motor complications with levodopa treatment, with a DA agonist unless congnitive or psychiatric problems were present or the degree of disability was severe enough as to require rapid therapeutic response. Limitations of DA agonists as monotherapy are that they may provide inadequate benefit, usually take longer than levodopa to reach effective doses, induce more early side effects and almost always require supplementary levodopa for control of disability after varying periods of time. DA agonists are also much more expensive than levodopa. DA agonists should not be used as first line therapy in elderly patients or in those with cognitive or psychiatric problems, in whom starting treatment with levodopa seems more appropiate.

Hallucinations and other drug induced psychotic states

Psychosis in untreated PD patients is rare (Factor et al., 1995) but in patients treated chronically with dopaminergic drugs, psychiatric symptoms are common and may affect to 10 to 50% of patients (Goodwin, 1971; Moskovitz, 1978; Rinne, 1983; Wilson and Smith, 1989). Psychiatric states can be induced or aggravated by most drugs given to PD patients, including levodopa, amantadine, selegiline or anticholinergics but the drugs with the highest potential to induce these side effects are the DA agonists.

Drug-induced psychosis can present with a wide clinical spectrum from occasional hallucinations to a full blown delirium. Benign organic hallucinosis with a normal state of consciousness is the most common mental side effect associated with dopaminergic therapy (Factor et al., 1995). Drug induced psychosis with altered sensorium is considered to be the most troublesome psychiatric symptom and is a frequent reason for nursing home placement of PD patients (Goetz et al., 1993). It causes more stress for care givers than does motor dysfunction. Mental aberrations induced by drugs occur more frequently in demented patients, in those exposed to high doses of dopamine agonists, in patients with premorbid psychiatric illness, and in the elderly. Combination therapy of levodopa with other medications is much more likely to cause confusional states (for review see Factor et al., 1995).

Treatment of psychiatric sympoms that accompany PD though poses a great challenge. On the one hand attempts to reduce or discontinue the offending drugs is met with reemergence of frequently unacceptable disabling motor symptoms. On the other hand the administration of conventional antipsychotics succesfully eliminates psychotic symptoms but also consistently worsens parkinsonsim. The complexities of these problem are particularly evident in PD patients with dementia in whom both parkinsonism and behavioural symptoms are disabling from the early stages and treating one aspect of the illness frequenly leads to deterioration of the other.

In the past decade a partial solution to this problem has been possible with the use of *atypical neuroleptics* to treat hallucination and psychosis in PD. Atypical antipsychotic drugs are characterized by less DA D2 receptor antagonism and more serotonine 5-HT2-receptor antagonism than classic neuroleptic drugs (Meltzer et al., 1989; Meltzer, 1993; Borison, 1995). The lower D2-receptor occupancy or the altered balance betweeen dopaminergic and serotonergic antagonism results in preserved or improved antipsychotic potency, with a reduction in extrapyramidal symptoms such as parkinsonism. The most effective atypical neuroleptic in the treatment of psychosis in PD is *clozapine* (Ostergard and Dupond, 1988; Friedman and Lannon, 1989; Lew, 1993; Gerlach and Peacock, 1994). This drug has revolutionized the management of avanced PD since it rarery worsens parkinsonsim and is highly effective in controlling psychosis. In contrast to the high doses of clozapine needed to control psychosis in schizophrenia very low doses of this drug are used in PD to succesfully manage hallucinations and other mental aberrations (Factor and Brown, 1992; Factor et al., 1994; Factor and Friedman, 1997; Fernandez and Durso, 1998; Pfeiffer et al., 1990; Trosch et al., 1998). The mean dose used in two double blind studies was 25 mg a day. Clozapine has also mild antiparkinsonian effects and has been reported to improve tremor and motor fluctuations. Side effects of clozapine include sedation, excessive salivation and postural hypotention. Unfortunatley its use has been associated to a 1% risk of inducing agranulocytosis (Krupp and Barnes, 1992), which makes regular frequent determinations of white counts necessary during its use.

Other atypical neuroleptics recently evaluated in the management of psychosis in PD include risperidone (Borison et al., 1992; Megens et al., 1994) and olanzapine (Moore et al., 1992). All reports on *risperidone* have been open label. In the initial report by Meco et al. (1994) all patients mental status improved without changes on the UPDRS. Subsequent studies though have shown worsening in parkinsonism in a high proportion of treated patients (Ford et al., 1994; Livingston, 1994; Rich et al., 1995; Workman et al., 1997). Furthermore questions concerning the "atypicality" of risperidone have been raised and tardive dyskinesias have been observed in two naive patients on risperidone. Therefore most clinicians do not advocate the use of these drug in PD. *Olanzapine* was the third atypical antipsychotic approved in the United States. It is more atypical than risperidone but less so than clozapine and does not have the risk of agranulocytosis. Although some open label studies have suggested that olanzapine can improve the mental status of PD patients without worsening parkinsonism (Wolters et al., 1997) a number of contrary reports have subsequently appeared (Friedman et al., 1998; Friedman, 1998; Aarsland et al., 1999; Graham et al., 1998); A randomized, double-blind parallel comparison of olanzapine (mean peak dose of 11 mg) and clozapine (mean peak dose 25 mg) in patients with PD with chronic hallucinations showed that at the doses used olanzapine aggravates parkinsonism in comparison with clozapine (Goetz et al., 2000). Manson et al. have also tested low dose olanzapine in the treatment of levodopa induced dyskinesias. They showed that the drug reduces dyskinesias in PD but even with the low doses used (1.25 to 7.25 mg/day) unacceptable increases in parkinsonism and "off" time occured. These agent should therefore not be regularly used in the management of hallucinations in patients with PD.

Recently *quetiapine* a dibenzo-thiazepine that blocks not only D1 and D2 receptors but also 5-HT1A and 5-HT2 receptors has been also found to have a beneficial effect in PD patients with hallucinations as described previousy with the other atypical neuroleptics (Parsa et al., 1998). Fernandez et al. (1999) reported on the use of quetiapine in 35 patients with drug induced psychosis. 20 of the 24 neuroleptic naive patients reported marked improvement of psychosis without a decline in motor function. In 11 psychiatrically stable patients on clozapine or olanzapine these investigators also tried to switch them to quetiapine but in six of these patients confusion and increased hallucinations occured. Weiner et al. (2000) reported a patient with levodopa-induced psychotic behaviour who did not respond well to olanzapine because of substantial worsening of motor function at very low doses but who was treated succesfully with quetiapine. In PD patients with psychosis treated with quetiapine Dewey and O'Suilleabhain (2000) reported an overall favorable response rate of 66%. Those patients that did not tolerate quetiapine or did not attain sufficent improvement were eventually well controlled with clozapine. There was no need to reduce dopaminergic drugs as the first step in the managemnt of psychosis. Quetiapine was easy to titrate on an outpatient bases and initiation of therapy was even possible by phone order to the pharmacy. Brandstater and Oertel (2002) have also presented data suporting the conclusion that quetiapine is an effcicient antipsychotic drug for the treatment of psychosis in the majority of patients with PD and its use does not requiere adaptation of antiparkinson drugs. There was no evidence of motor worsening in either study which included 25 patients.

From the available data it can be concluded that quetipine is usefull and well tolerated as a first drug to treat drug induced psychosis in PD (Matheson and Lamb, 2000). It rarely causes increse in parkinsonisms (Fernandez, 2000) and is not associated with agranulocytosis. It must be used cautiously to replace other atypical neuroleptic drugs in patients with well controlled psychiatric symptoms.

Ondansetron is a serotonin 5-HT3 receptor antagonist used with success in schizophrenic patients at doses of 12–20 mg/day (White et al., 1991). Extrapyramidal side effects are extremely rare, however, dystonia and akathisia were described in neoplasic patients on chemotherapy receiving ondansetron as antiemetic therapy (Halperin and Murphy, 1992). In a study on seven parkinsonian patients with hallucinations induced by dopaminergic therapy, ondansetron was effective in all, reducing the symptomatology in four of them and abolishing hallucinations in three (Zoldan et al., 1993). Discontinuation of the drug resulted in reappearance of symptoms in a few days. No adverse side effects were described. In another study by the same author, 16 parkinsonian patients with psychotic symptoms, treated with levodopa, received increasing doses of ondansetron escalated by 4 to 8 mg per week up to a total maintenance dose of 12 to 24 mg/day. Ondansetron did not worsen the motor features or interefered with levodopa efficacy. In addition, hallucinations, paranoid delusions and other psychotic symptoms improved markedly in most of patients on this study (Zoldan et al., 1996). Adverse effects consisting on occasional headaches and aggravation of constipation in a few patients, were mild. Further studies will be needed to ascertain these optimistic findings.

The efficacy of the pure serotonin blockers, such as ondansetron, in the treatment of hallucinosis in PD might be produced by inhibition of corticolimbic serotonergic receptors in drug-induced psychosis. It has been suggested that these receptors are overstimulated by serotonin flushed out of nerve terminals by extraordinary high cerebrospinal dopamine levels (Nausieda et al., 1983).

Treatment of cognitive impairment in Parkinson disease

In PD specific cognitive areas, such as visuospatial function, certain forms of memory and executive functions, are commonly altered. Such cognitive abnormalities not amounting to dementia may occur, according to some series, in almost all patients. PD patients have also increased risk for becoming demented compared with subjets without PD (Aarsland et al., 2001). Prevalence estimates of dementia range from 4 to 93%. Methodological differences among studies probably account for these discrepant estimates. Overall, among recent, methodologically sounder studies, the average prevalence falls into the 25–30% range. Since patients with PD and dementia (PDD) die sooner than those non demented patients current prevalence estimates might underestimate the frequency of dementia in PD.

The neuropathological substrate of dementia in PD is unclear. It has been attributed to concomitant Alzheimer disease since some postmortem studies of patients with PD dementia shown changes consistent with PD plus changes indistinguishable from those typically found in Alzheimer disease (Hakim and Mathieson, 1979; Boller et al., 1980; Quinn et al., 1986). However some studies have not found and association between PD dementia and Alzheimer disease (Tagliavini et al., 1984; Rinne et al., 1989). Some authors have attributed dementia in PD primarily to loss of neurons in the medial part of the substantia nigra (Rinne et al., 1989) and still others to degeneration in various combinations of subcortical nuclei such as the cholinergic nucleus basalis (Perry et al., 1995), the locus ceruleus (Cash et al., 1987; Zweig et al., 1993) and the raphe nucleus.

Recent studies, using newer inmunohistochemichal techniques that allow for an easier detection of Lewy bodies (LB), have described demented parkinsonian patients in whom widespread LB are present in the cerebral cortex (Lenox et al., 1989; Hansen et al., 1990; Hurtig et al., 2000) and have suggested that the presence of diffuse cortical Lewy bodies (CLB) are a more sensitive and specific correlate of dementia in PD than the presence of Alzheimer pathlogy (Calopa et al., 2002).

The clinical and neuropathological similarities between dementia with Lewy bodies (DLB) and Parkinson disease dementia on the one hand and the recently described favorable response of DLB to the cholinesterase inhibitors has suggested that these drugs could be of benefit in the management of the dementia in PD. In addition, in patients with PD and dementia an important subcortical cholinergic deficit has been described. In DLB rivastigmine (McKeith et al., 2000) improved symptoms such as anxiety and apathy, impaired attention, unresponsiveness and daytime somnolence. Patients, furthermore, had fewer delusions and hallucinations. Objective measures of cognition, especially memory and attention also improved.

Information on the use of cholinesterase inhibitors in PD is sparse but results seem promising. Tacrine was used and appeared usefull (Hutchinson and Fazzini, 1996). It was encouraging to notice that with cholinesterase inhibitors motor function did not worsen in PD patients. A more recent open label report on the use of rivastigmine in PD has appeared (Reading et al., 2002). In this study the ability of rivastigmine to treat the neuropsychiatric complications of advanced PD was assesed in 12 patients. Hallucinations, sleep disturbance and carer distress were all improved and cognitive performance enhanced. In any case did motor scores worsen. These results are similar to those found in studies using comparable asessments of patients diagnosed with DLB.

Level-I trials of several cholinesterase inhibitors in PD are in progress. The use of these drugs, though, provides a new approach to a difficult clinical problem. It also emphazises the potential importance of cholinergic mechanisms in the neuropsychiatric complications or neurodegenerative disorders (Reading et al., 2002).

References

Aarsland D, Larsen JP, Lim NG, Tandberg E (1999) Olanzapine for psychosis in patients with Parkinson's disease with and without dementia. J Neuropsychiatry Clin Neurosci 11: 392–394

Aarsland D, Andersen K, Larsen JP, Lolk A, Nielsen H, Kragh-Sorensen (2001) Risk of dementia in Parkinson's disease. A community-based, prospective study. Neurology 56: 730–736

Adler CH, Sethi KD, Hauser RA, et al (1997) Ropinirole for the treatment of early Parkinson's disease. Neurology 49: 393–399

Adler CH, Singer C, O'Brien C, hauser RA, Lew MF, Marek KL, et al (1998) Randomized, placebo-controlled study of tolcapone in patients with fluctuating Parkinson's disease treated with levodopa-carbidopa. Arch Neurol 55: 421–428
Agid Y, Ahlskog A, Albanese A, et al (1999) Levodopa in the treatment of Parkinson's disease: a consensus meeting. Mov Disord 14: 911–913
Boller F, Mizutani T, Roessmann U, Gambetti P (1980) Parkinsons disease, dementia and Alzheimer disease: clinicopathological correlations. Ann Neurol 7: 329–335
Borison RL (1995) Clinical efficacy of serotonin-dopamine antagonists relative to classic neuroleptics. J Clin Psychopharmacol 15 [Suppl 1]: 24–29
Borison RL, Rathiraja AP, Bruce I, et al (1992) Risperidone: clinical safety and efficacy in schizophrenia. Psychopharmacol Bull 28: 213–218
Brandstäder D, Oertel WH (2002) Treatment of drug-induced psychosis with quetiapine and clozapine in Parkinson's disease. Neurology 58: 160–161
Calopa M, Tolosa E, Ferrer I, et al (2002) In: Tolosa E, Schultz J, McKeith I, Ferrer I (eds) Neurodegenerative disorders asociated with alpha synuclein pathology. Medicina STM Editores, Barcelona, pp 127–135
Cash R, Donnis T, L'Heureux R, Raisman R, Javoy-Agid F, Scatton B (1987) Parkinson's disease and dementia: norepinephrine and dopamine in locus ceruleus. Neurology 37: 42–46
Cotzias GC, Van Woert MH, Schiffer LM (1970) Aromatic amino acids and modification of parkinsonism. N Engl J Med 282: 31–33
Dewey RB, O'Suilleabhain PE (2000) Treatment of drug-induced psychosis with quetiapine and clozapine in Parkinson's disease. Neurology 55: 1753–1754
Factor SA, Brown D (1992) Clozapine prevents recurrence of psychosis in Parkinson's disease. Mov Disord 7: 125–131
Factor SA, Friedman JH (1997) The emerging role of clozapine in the treatment of movement disorders. Mov Disord 12: 483–496
Factor SA, Brown D, Molho ES, Podskalny GD (1994) Clozapine: a 2-year open trial in PD patients with psychosis. Neurology 44: 544–546
Factor SA, Molho ES, Podskalny GD, Brown D (1995) Parkinson's disease: drug-induced psychiatric states. In: Weiner WJ, Lang AE (eds) Advances in neurology, vol 65. Raven Press, New York, pp 115–138
Fahn S (1974) On-off phenomenon with levodopa therapy in parkinsonism. Neurology 24: 431–441
Fernández HH (2000) Quetiapine for l-dopa induced psychosis in PD. Neurology 55: 899
Fernandez HH, Durso R (1998) Clozapine for dopaniergic-induced paraphilias in Parkinson's disease. Mov Disord 13: 597–598
Fernández HH, Friedman JH, Jacques C, Rosenfeld M (1999) Quetiapine for the treatment of drug-induced psychosis in Parkinson's disease. Mov Disord 14: 484–487
Friedman JH (1998) Olanzapine in the treatment of dopaminomimetic psychosis in patients with Parkinson's disease. Neurology 50: 1195–1196
Friedman JH, Lannon MC (1989) Clozapine in the treatment of psychosis in PD. Neurology 39: 1219–1221
Friedman JH, Goldstein S, Jacques C (1998) Substituting clozapine for olanzapine in psychiatrically stable Parkinson's disease patients: results of an open label pilot study. Clin Neuropharmacol 5: 285–288
Gerlach J, Peacock L (1994) Motor and mental side effects of clozapine. J Clin Psychiatry 55 [Suppl B]: S107–S109
Goetz C (1998) Influence of COMT inhibition on levodopa pharmacology and therapy. Neurology 50 [Suppl 5]: 26–30
Goetz CG, Stebbins GT (1993) Risk factors for nursing home placement in advanced Parkinson's disease. Neurology 43: 2227–2229
Goetz CG, Vogel C, Tanner CM, Stebbins GT (1998) Early dopaminergic drug-induced hallucinations in parkinsonian patients. Neurology 51: 811–814

Goetz CG, Blasucci LM, Leurgans S, Pappert EJ (2000) Olanzapine and clozapine. Comparative effects on motor function in hallucinating PD patients. Neurology 55: 748–749
Goodwin FK (1971) Psychiatric side effects of l-dopa in man. JAMA 218: 1915–1920
Graham JM, Sussman JD, Ford KS, Sagar HJ (1998) Olanzapine in the treatment of hallucinosis in idiopathic Parkinson's disease: a cautionary note. J Neurol Neurosurg Pschiatry 65: 774–777
Hakim A, Mathieson G (1979) Dementia in Parkinson disease: a neuropathologic study. Neurology 29: 1209–1214
Halperin JR, Murphy B (1992) Extrapyramidal reaction to ondansetron. Cancer 69: 1275
Hansen L, Salmon D, Galasko D, Masliah E, Katzman R, De Teresa R, Thal L, Pay MM, Hofstetter R, Klauber M, Rice V, Butters N, Alford M (1990) The Lewy body variant of Alzheimer's disease: a clinical and pathologic entity. Neurology 40: 1–8
Hurtig HI, Trojanowski JQ, Galvin J, Ewbank D, Schmidt ML, Lee VM-Y, Clark CM, Glosser G, Stern MB, Gollomp SM, Arnold SE (2000) α-synuclein cortical Lewy bodies correlate with dementia in Parkinson's disease. Neurology 54: 1916–1921
Hutchinson M, Fazzini E (1996) Cholinesterase inhibition in Parkinson's disease. J Neurol Neurosurg Psychiatry 61: 324–325
Keränen T, Gordin A, Harjola VP, Karlsson M, Korpela K, y cols (1996) The effect of cathecol-O-methyltransferase inhibition by entacapone on the pharmacokinetics and metabolism of levodopa in healthy volunteers. Clin Neuropharmacol 50: 47–55
Kieburtz K, Shoulson I, McDermontt M, et al (1997) Safety and efficacy of pramipexole, in early Parkinson disease. A randomized dose-ranging study. JAMA 278: 125–130
Klawans HL (1986) Individual manifestations of Parkinson's disease after ten or more years of levodopa. Mov Disord 1: 187–192
Krupp P, Barnes P (1992) Clozapine-associated agranulocytosis: risk and aetiology. Br J Psychiatry 160 [Suppl 17]: 38–40
Kurth MC, Adler CH (1998) COMT inhibition: a new strategy for Parkinson's disease. Neurology 50 [Suppl 5]: 3–14
Kuruma I, Bartholini G, Tissot R, Pletscher A (1971) The metabolism of L-3-Omethyldopa, a precursor in man. Clin Pharmacol Ther 12: 678–682
Lennox G, Lowe J, Morrell K, Landon M, Mayer RJ (1989) Anti-ubiquitin immunocytochemistry is more sensitive than conventional techniques in the detection of diffuse Lewy body disease. J Neurol Neusosurg Psychiatry 52: 67–71
Lew MF, Waters CH (1993) Clozapine treatment of parkinsonism with psychosis. J Am Geriatr Soc 41: 669–671
Livingston MG (1994) Risperidone. Lancet 343: 457–460
Männistö PT (1994) Clinical potential of catechol-O-methyltransferase (COMT) inhibitors as adjuvants in Parkinson's disease. CNS Drugs 1: 172–179
Männistö PT, Kaakkola S (1989) New selective COMT inhibitors: useful adjuncts for Parkinson's disease? Trends Pharmacol Sci 10: 47–55
Männistö PT, Tuomainen P, Tuomainen PK (1992) Different in vivo properties of three new inhibitors of cathechol-O-methyl transferase in rat. Br J Pharmacol 105: 569–574
Manson AJ, Schrag A, Lees AJ (2000) Low-dose olanzapine for levodopa induced dyskinesias. Neurology 55: 795–799
Marsden CD, Parkes JP, Quinn N (1982) Fluctuations of disability in Parkinson's disease. In: Marsden CD, Fahn S (eds) Movement disorders. Butterworth, London
Matheson AJ, Lamb HM (2000) Quetiapine. A review of its clinical potential in the management of psychotic symptoms in Parkinson's disease. CNS Drugs 14: 157–172
McKeith I, Del Ser T, Spano P, Emre M, Wesnes K, Anand R, Cicin-Sain A (2000) Efficacy of rivastigmine in dementia with Lewy bodies: a randomized, double-blind, placebo-controlled international study. Lancet 356: 2031–2036
Meco G, Alessandria A, Binfati V, Giustini P (1994) Risperidone for hallucinations in l-dopa-treated PD patients. Lancet 343: 1370–1371

Megens AAHP, Awouters FHL, Schotte A, et al (1994) Survey on the pharmacodynamics of the new antipsychotic risperidone. Psychopharmacol 114: 9–23
Meltzer HY (1993) New drugs for the treatment of schizophrenia. Psychiatr Clin North Am 16: 365–385
Meltzer HY, Matsubara S, Lee J-C (1989) Classification of typical and atypical antipsychotic drugs on the basis of dopamine D1, D2 and serotonin-2 pKi values. J Pharmacol Exp Ther 251: 238–246
Moore NA, Tye NC, Axton MS, Risius FC (1992) The behavioural pharmacology of olanzapine, a novel "atypical" antipsychotic agent. J Pharmacol Exp Ther 262: 545–551
Moskovitz C, Moses H, Klawans H (1978) L-dopa induced psychosis: a kindling phenomena. Am J Psychiatry 135: 6–10
Nausieda P, Tanner C, Klawans H (1983) Serotonergically active agents in the treatment of the l-dopa induced psychosis. In: Fahn S, Calne DB, Shoulson I (eds) Experimental therapeutics of movement disorders. Raven Press, New York, pp 23–32 (Adv Neurol 37)
Nutt JG, Fellman JH (1984) Pharmacokinetics of levodopa. Clin Neuropharmacol 7: 35–49
Nutt JC (1990) Levodopa induced dyskinesia. Neurology 40: 340–345
Ostergaard K, Dupond E (1988) Clozapine treatment of drug-induced psychotic symptoms in late stages of PD. Acta Neurol Scand 78: 349–350
Papavasiliou PS, Cotzias GC, Duby SE, et al (1972) Levodopa in parkinsonism: potentiation of central effets with a peripheral inhibitor. N Engl J Med 285: 8–14
Parkinson Study Group (1997) Entacapone improves motor fluctuations in levodopa-treated Parkinson's disease patients. Ann Neurol 4 [Suppl 3]: 3–11
Parkinson Study Group (1999) Low-dose clozapine for the treatment of drug-induced psychosis in Parkinson's disease. N Engl J Med 340: 757–763
Parkinson Study Group (2000) Pramipexole vs levodopa as initial treatment for Parkinson's disease. JAMA 284: 1931–1938
Parsa MA, Bastani B (1998) Quetiapine (Seroquel) in the treatment of psychosis in patients with Parkinson's disease. J Neuropsychiatry Clin Neurosci 10: 216–219
Perry EK, Curtis M, Dick DJ, Candy JM, Atack JR, Bloxham CA, Blessed G, Fairbairn A, Tomlinson BE, Perry RM (1985) Cholinergic correlates of cognitive impairment in Parkinson's disease: comparisons with Alzheimer's disease. J Neurol Neurosurg Psychiatry 48: 413–421
Perry RH, Irving D, Blessed G, Perry EK, Fairbairn A (1989) Senile dementia of Lewy body type and spectrum of Lewy body disease Lancet i: 1088
Pfeiffer RF, Kang J, Graber B, Hofman R, Wilson J (1990) Clozapine for psychosis in Parkinson's disease. Mov Disord 5: 239–242
Quinn NP, Rossor MN, Marsden CD (1986) Dementia and Parkinson's disease: pathological and neurochemical consequences. Br Med Bull 42: 86–90
Rajput AH, Martin W, Saint-Hilaire MH, Dorflinger E, Pedder S (1997) Tolcapone improves motor function in parkinsonian patients with the "wearing-off" phenomenon: a double-blind, placebo-controlled, multicenter trial. Neurology 49: 1066–1071
Rascol A, Montastruc JL, Guirard-Chaumeil B, Clanet M (1982) Bromocriptine as first treatment of Parkinson's disease. Long-term results. Rev Neurol 138: 402–408
Rascol O, Brooks DJ, Korczyn AD, et al (2000) A five-year study of the incidence of dyskinesia in patients with early Parkinson's disease who were treated with ropinirole or levodopa. N Engl J Med 342: 1484–1491
Reading PJ, et al (2001) Rivastigmine in the treatment of parkinsonian psychosis and cognitive impairment: preliminary findings from an open trial. Mov Disord 16: 1171–1195
Rich SS, Friedman JH, Ott BR (1995) Risperidone versus clozapine in the treatment of psychosis in six patients with Parkinson's disease and other akinetic-rigid syndromes. J Clin Psychiatry 56: 556–559

Rinne JO, Rummukainen J, Paijarvi L, Rinne UK (1989) Dementia in Parkinson's disease is related to neuronal loss in the medial substantia nigra. Ann Neurol 25: 146–151

Rinne UK (1983) Problems associated with long term levodopa treatment of Parkinson's disease. Acta Neurol Scand 95: 19–26

Rinne UK, Bracco F, Chouza C, et al (1997) Cabergoline in the treatment of early Parkinson's disease: results of the first year of treatment in a double-blind comparison of cabergoline and levodopa. Neurology 48: 363–368

Rinne UK, Bracco F, Chouza C, et al (1998) Early treatment of Parkinson's disease with cabergoline delays the onset of motor complications. Results of a double-blind levodopa controlled trial. The PkDS009 study Group. Drugs 55 [Suppl 1]: 23–30

Rinne UK, Larsen JP, Siden A, Worm-Petersen J (1998) The Nomecomt Study Group. Entacapone enhances the response to levodopa in Parkinsonian patients with motor fluctuations. Neurology 51: 1309–1314

Sánchez-Ramos JR (1997) High dose pergolide monotherapy for the treatment of severe dyskinesias in Parkinson's disease. In: Olanow WC, Obeso JA (eds) Beyond the decade of the brain, vol 2. Dopamine agonists in early Parkinson's disease. Wells Medical Limited, UK, pp 217–232

Sethi KD, O'Brien CF, Hammerstad JP, et al (1998) Ropinirole for the treatment of early Parkinson's disease- a 12-month experience. Arch Neurol 55: 1211–1216

Shannon KM, Bennett JP Jr., Friedman JH (1997) Efficacy of pramipexole, a novel dopamine agonist, as monotherapy in mild to moderate Parkinson's disease. Neurology 49: 724–728

Tagliavini F, Pilleri G, Bouras C, Constantinidis J (1992) The basal nucleus of Meynert in idiopathic Parkinson's disease. Acta Neurol Scand 69: 20–28

Tolosa E (1998) Current Parkinson's disease therapy. Levodopa-The Gold Standard. Clin Neuropharmacol 21 [Suppl 1]: S1–S4

Tolosa E (1999) Levodopa-induced dyskinesias and fluctuations in Parkinson disease. PIL, París

Tolosa E, Marin C (1997) Dopamine agonists in Parkinson's disease: a clinical review. In: Olanow WC, Obeso JA (eds) Beyond the decade of the brain, vol 2. Dopamine agonists in early Parkinson's disease. Wells Medical Limited, UK, pp 143–161

Tolosa E, Martín W, Cohen H, Jacobson J (1975) Patterns of clinical response and plasma dopa levels in Parkinson's disease. Neurology 25(2): 177–183

Tolosa E, Blesa R, Bayes A, et al (1987) Low-dose bromocriptine in early phases of Parkinson's disease. Clin Neuropharmacol 10: 169–174

Tolosa E, Valldeoriola F, Martí MJ (1994) New and emerging strategies for improving levodopa treatment. Neurology 44: 535–544

Trosch RM, Friedman JH, Lannon MC, Pahwa R, Smith D, Seeberger LC, O'Brien CF, LeWitt PA, Koller WC (1998) Clozapine use in Parkinson's disease: a retrospective analysis of a large multicentered clinical experience. Mov Disord 13: 377–382

Weiner WJ, Minagar A, Shulman LM (2000) Quetiapine for l-dopa induced psychosis in PD. Neurology 54: 1538

White A, Corn TH, Feetham, Faulconbridge C (1991) Ondansetron in treatment of schizophrenia. Lancet 337: 1173

Wilson JA, Smith RG (1989) The prevalence and aetiology of long term L-dopa side effects in elderly parkinsonian patients. Age Ageing 18: 11–16

Wolters EC, Hurwitz TA, Mak E, et al (1990) Clozapine in the treatment of parkinsonian patients with dopaminomimetic psychosis. Neurology 40: 832–834

Wolters EC, Jansen EN, Tuynman-Qua HG, Bergmans PL (1997) Olanzapine in the treatment of dopaminomimetic psychosis in patients with Parkinson's disease. Neurology 47: 1085–1087

Workman RH Jr, Orengo CA, Bakey AA, Molinari VA, Kunik ME (1997) The use of risperidone for psychosis and agitation in demented patients with PD. J Neuropsychiatry Clin Neurosci 9: 594–597

Zoldan J, Friedberg G, Goldberg-Stern, Melamed E (1993) Ondansentron for hallucinosis in advanced Parkinson's disease. Lancet 341: 562–563
Zoldan J, Friedberg G, Weizman A, Melamed E (1996) Ondansetron, a 5-HT3 antagonist for visual hallucinations and paranoid delusional disorder associated with chronic L-DOPA therapy in advanced Parkinson's disease. In: Battistin L, Scarlato G, Caraceni T, Ruggieri S (eds) Parkinson's disease. Lippincot-Raven, Philadelphia, pp 541–544 (Adv Neurol 69)
Zweig RM, Cardillo JE, Cohen M, Giere S, Hedreen JC (1993) The locus ceruleus and dementia in Parkinson's disease. Neurology 43: 986–991

Author's address: E. Tolosa, M.D., Neurology Service, ICMSN, and Banco de Tejidos Neurológicos, Hospital Clinico, University of Barcelona, Villaroel 170, E-080036 Barcelona, Spain, e-mail: etolosa@clinic.ub.es

J Neural Transm (2003) [Suppl] 64: 79–93

Depression and antisocial personality disorder: two contrasting disorders of 5HT function

J. F. W. Deakin

Neuroscience and Psychiatry Unit, University of Manchester, United Kingdom

Summary. Impaired 5HT functioning has been implicated in two very different psychiatric syndromes: antisocial personality disorder and depression. In both, reduced csf concentration of 5HIAA and blunted circulating hormone responses to 5HT drug challenge have been described. The paradox can be resolved by the theory that the two main ascending 5HT pathways mediate adaptive responses to future and current adversity. Projections of the anterior group of raphe 5HT cells (dorsal raphe nucleus) oppose the action of dopamine and mediate avoidance of threats. Impaired function sensitises the dopamine system resulting in impulsivity and drug addiction. Posterior 5HT cells (median raphe nucleus) innervate hippocampus and cingulate gyrus and suppress memory and awareness of current and past adversity. Impaired function results in low mood, low self-esteem, hopelessness and pessimism. Modern imaging methods are providing startling corroboration of these ideas.

Introduction

5-HT has been implicated in most psychiatric disorders: Alzheimer's disease, attention deficit disorder and alcoholism just to mention three that begin with "A". If there were psychiatric disorders that begin with X, Y or Z, it is likely that a 5-HT aetiology would have been proposed. It very apposite that I am discussing 5HT in 2002 as this is the 50th anniversary of its discovery in brain.

In this talk I will focus on two disorders for which there is the most consistent evidence for an impairment of 5-HT function. They are impulsive, aggressive personality disorders on the one hand and depression on the other. Impulsivity, aggression, psychopathy, arson and drug abuse have all been associated with a so-called low 5-HT syndrome [1]. On the other hand, much evidence is compatible with the idea that depression results from defective 5-HT neurotransmission in the brain and yet the symptoms could not be more different from personality disorder [2]. They include depressed mood, anxiety, panic neuro-vegetative changes including loss of appetite and insomnia. Suicidal ideation and acts are common. For both disorders, the same kind of biological abnormalities have been claimed. There are well over 100 studies of the csf 5-HT metabolite 5HIAA concentrations in depression, many of which report decreases compared with controls. However, the findings are by no means unanimous and there are a number of negative findings. There have been fewer studies of csf in patients with personality disorder but they all report reductions in relation to impulsivity or aggression.

CSF 5HIAA concentration is a static measure of 5HT turnover. Drugs with actions on 5HT systems have been used as probes of dynamic 5HT function. For example, fenfluramine releases 5HT which in turn induces increases in pituitary secretion of prolactin and ACTH, and the latter causes increases in circulating cortisol concentration. The magnitude of hormone responses is taken as a measure of dynamic 5HT function [3]. In personality disorders a number of studies report reduced prolactin responses to the 5-HT releasing agent, fenfluramine, and after m-chlorophenylpiperazine (mCPP) which acts directly on 5HT receptors.

Attenuated hormonal responses to fenfluramine have been claimed in depression. However, the literature is quite contradictory with some studies reporting attenuated responses in sub-groups of depressed patients, but larger group comparisons of depressives vs controls find no change or even increases. Evidence for blunting of hormonal responses in depression has been more consistent when the 5-HT precursor, tryptophan has been used to probe 5HT function [4]. Studies with this challenge have not been reported in personality disorders. The fact that depression responds to treatment with serotonin specific re-uptake inhibitors is compatible with the idea that these drugs work by reversing an impairment of 5-HT functioning in the disorder. It is much less clear whether SSRIs are effective in the treatment of antisocial personality disorder despite much speculation in this possibility [5].

In this talk I will investigate the question of what the normal behavioural functions of 5-HT are in an attempt to understand how impaired 5HT function could give rise to very different clinical manifestations. I will highlight findings in humans with new imaging methods.

Discovery of serotonin

Serotonin was discovered in the brain 50 years ago — exactly 50 years ago from the British perspective. A good account may be found in Whitaker-Azmitia [6] although the British contribution is perhaps neglected. In 1952 Amin and Crawford [7] presented an oral communication to the British Physiological Society on the extraction of 5-hydroxytryptamine and substance P from the brain. The first publication, however, was in 1953 by Twarog and Page who also isolated (5-HT but not substance P) in brain samples and other organs of the body. Amin and Crawford did not publish their findings until 1954 [7]. Soon after these publications, Woolley and Shaw proposed that 5-HT might have a role in mental illness particularly psychosis because LSD antagonised some of the effects of 5-HT on vaso-constriction. In 1957 Gaddum and Piccarelli deduced that there must be at least two kinds of 5-HT receptors. We now know there are at least seven families and each family has a number of sub-types. In 1965 Dahlstrom and Fuxe made the first visualisations of 5-HT in the brain [8]. Sections were exposed to formaldehyde vapour which reacted with serotonin to form a fluorescent compound. Using a fluorescence microscope, brightly fluorescent 5-HT containing cells and fibres could be visualised against the dark background of the rest of the brain stem. They described a number of groups of 5-HT containing cells in the midline, raphe, of the brainstem.

Studies by Dahlstrom and Fuxe showed that the 5-HT system was incredibly divergent. Cell bodies were localised in the brainstem and from relatively small numbers, the entire forebrain was innervated with a fine net of diffusively branching axons and terminals. At least four different pathways have been described in the rodent ascending from the raphe nuclei and I think that two of them are particularly relevant to today's issue; 5-HT deficiency in different pathways innervating different parts of the brain may give rise to different clinical pictures.

The dorsal raphe nucleus lies under the aqueduct which connects the fourth ventricle to the third ventricle. It is about 2.5 cm in anterior-posterior extent and contains about a quarter of a million neurones [9]. 165,000 of them contain serotonin and of those, 75,000 also contain the peptide, substance P. It is interesting that both these compounds should have been isolated by Amin and Crawford. About 5,000 dorsal raphe neurones contain dopamine but they do not contain 5-HT and they are located at the anterior end of the dorsal raphe nucleus. From this very small nucleus and its small number of cells relative to the millions of cells in the forebrain, arises the highly divergent system of 5-HT fibres. It is remarkable that modern imaging techniques have been able to visualise this small brainstem nucleus in living human subjects. For example, Morris et al. [10] observed increased metabolic activity within the dorsal raphe nucleus in depressed patients whose circulating tryptophan concentrations had been severely decreased by a technique which I will describe later. In their paper, the dorsal raphe nucleus can be clearly seen lying beneath the cerebral aqueduct. Their explanation was that the cells in the nucleus were being activated by a negative feedback system in response to the lack of serotonin in terminal regions caused by depletion of tryptophan.

Functional anatomy of two ascending 5HT projections; overview

Different groups of 5-HT containing cells within the raphe, project to different forebrain areas. In this talk I will suggest that the two 5-HT deficiency disorders maybe understood in terms of dysfunction in two distinct 5-HT systems [11]. It is well known that cells of the dorsal raphe nucleus project to dopaminergic structures while cells in the median raphe nucleus project to hippocampus more in parallel with noradrenergic nerve terminals [12, 13, 14]. Studies by Imai [12] clearly indicate that the true distinction between the dorsal and the median raphe nucleus may also be understood in terms of an anterior-posterior distinction. In this retrograde labelling study, two clear bands of 5-HT containing neurones were found to contain tracer dyes which had been retrogradely transported from injection sites in forebrain areas. The anterior band of raphe cells was retrogradely labelled following tracer injections in the caudate nucleus while the more posterior band was retrogradely labelled from injections in the hippocampus. In keeping with the parallelism between dopamine projections and the projections of the anterior group of 5-HT cells, it is the anterior group which project to the ventral tegmental area and the substantia nigra while the posterior group project to the noradrenergic locus coeruleus. The amygdala comprises several sub-nuclei and there are distinct noradrenergic and dopaminergic projections to them. Interestingly, both the anterior and posterior group of 5-HT cells project to amygdala.

Many studies indicate that 5-HT release is enhanced by aversive stimuli in various forebrain areas (see [11]). I suggested that anterior 5-HT containing cells in parallel with dopamine modulate forebrain systems concerned with locomotor guidance to home-in on positive incentive stimuli in the environment and to avoid aversive ones [15]. The anterior 5-HT system can thus be regarded as a system for keeping us out of trouble. In contrast, various lines of evidence suggest that posterior 5-HT cells projecting to hippocampus are concerned with adaptation to aversive stimuli once they have occurred [16]; a system for coping with trouble once it has occurred. This allows normal behaviour to re-emerge in the face of chronic aversion or 'stress'. I suggest that impulsive personality disorders can be seen as the result of a long-term failure of the anterior raphe anticipatory avoidance mechanism. In contrast, depression may arise from a failure of the posterior 5HT system resulting in failure of adaptation or tolerance to stress.

Antisocial personality disorder and the anterior 5-HT negative incentive system

Reward and dopamine mechanisms

A wealth of animal behavioural evidence suggests that the major function of dopamine is to mediate incentive motivation. The first lines of evidence came from the discovery of intra-cranial brain stimulation reward. In 1953, Olds and Milner demonstrated that rats would rapidly acquire lever pressing in order to stimulate the median forebrain bundle through chronically implanted electrodes [17]. Subsequent mapping studies showed a remarkable parallelism with the distribution of dopamine cell bodies, fibre tracts and terminals. Lesioning dopamine pathways with the specific catecholamine neurotoxin 6-hydroxydopamine and administration of dopamine receptor antagonists caused the behaviour to extinguish. The behaviour was dependent on intact mesolimbic dopaminergic projections [18]. Drugs of abuse share the ability to enhance dopamine release from mesolimbic terminals and this is thought to be the common mechanism of addiction [19].

Until recently it has not been possible to demonstrate this convincingly in humans. The advent of modern imaging techniques have proved a way forward. For example, Elliott et al. showed that a visual display of cumulative winnings in a guessing game correlated with the BOLD signal in the region of the substantia nigra and the dopaminergic cell bodies of the brain stem [20], detected using functional magnetic resonance imaging (fMRI). In addition activation was also seen in the ventral striatum and anterior cingulate and these areas are also richly innervated with dopamine. Using positron emission tomography, Koepp et al. demonstrated that successful performance in a computer game was associated with displacement of C11 raclopride binding to dopamine receptors in the ventral striatum [21]. This suggests that the reward increased the release of dopamine which displaced radioactive raclopride binding to dopamine receptors.

Aversion and the anterior 5HT negative-incentive system

Deakin [11, 15, 16] proposed that anterior dorsal raphe projections to accumbens, striatum and pre-frontal cortex are activated by aversive cues, that is, danger stimuli which predict a noxious or disadvantageous outcome. Many studies have shown that 5-HT release increases after aversive cues in terminal regions of the anterior 5-HT cells [22]. However, electrophysiological studies of raphe cells do not find major changes in firing rate in relation to stressful stimuli [23]. It may be that aversive stimuli increase 5HT release via other neurotransmitters such as glutamate acting on the 5HT terminal rather than by increasing firing rate of brainstem cell bodies. The behavioural effect of increased 5HT release in dopaminergic areas is to prevent further approach behaviour and to orient the animal away from aversive cues towards neutral or safety stimuli. These are approached through the action of the dopamine incentive system [15, 24].

Consequences of impaired anterior 5HT function

Removal of the 5HT stop system results in a failure to avoid risks and in excessive control of behaviours by rewards. These proposals are based on evidence from various 5HT manipulations in experimental animals. For example, normal animals trained to bar-press for food or water suppress responding when cues predict footshock. Animals depleted of forebrain 5HT (by neurotoxin lesions of 5-HT cells in the raphe or of terminals in the amygdala) are less able to suppress responding [25, 26] in the presence of footshock cues. Depletion of 5HT in the nucleus accumbens is associated with increased locomotor activity and an increased speed of responding for food reward in the 5-choice box task [27] and of impulsive premature responding (Harrison). Some of these effects were prevented by dopamine receptor blockade [28]. Normal animals will learn to press a lever that has no consequence other than to turn on a cue such as a light or tone previously paired with a reward such as water in thirsty animals (secondary reinforcement). 5HT-depleted animals show greater rates of lever pressing for secondary reinforcement [29].

Rocha et al. [30] showed a particularly dramatic consequence of interfering with this system by genetically engineering mice which lack the 5-HT1B receptor gene (5-HT1B receptor knockout mice). 5-HT1B receptor knockout mice lack 5HT restraint of dopamine systems. The detailed mechanism is unclear but 5-HT1B receptors are located on 5-HT terminals and on GABA cell bodies and terminals in ventral striatum and the ventral tegmental area. 5HT and GABA modify dopamine release in these areas. The knockout mice show enhanced locomotor responses to cocaine (dopamine releaser) and very impressive increases in bar pressing for intravenous self-administration of cocaine. Neurochemical studies indicate that the dopamine system is hyperactive in these animals. Furthermore, they are impulsive and aggressive in their general behaviour. This suggests a very novel and insightful explanation for the clinical association between impulsive personality disorders and addiction. The assumption has often been that impulsive personality traits increase risky behaviours including experimenting with drugs. The 5-HT1B knockout mouse suggests that both the impulsive behaviour and the tendency to addiction may have an underlying common mechanism namely sensitisation of forebrain dopaminergic projections. Thus impulsive individuals through impaired 5-HT functioning may have dopaminergic systems which are sensitised. This leads to impulsive behaviour on the one hand and to immediate and rapid addiction on the other.

5HT restraint of behaviour in man

Does 5-HT restrain behaviour in Man? We have used the technique of tryptophan depletion to investigate this question. Tryptophan is an amino-acid taken in the diet. It is the precursor of serotonin — 5HT is synthesised from it in 5HT neurones. In brief, the technique involves administration of a large oral load of amino acids excepting tryptophan. The ensuing protein synthesis in the liver incorporates tryptophan from the circulation and circulating levels decrease by up to 80%. Thus brain 5HT neurones are deprived of the precursor of 5HT this is associated with significant reductions in 5-HT release in the brain.

In a parallel group design, we compared subjects depleted of tryptophan with subjects who received a control drink containing tryptophan [31]. A highly significant 70% decrease in circulating tryptophan concentrations was seen in the depleted group. They carried out a variety of neuropsychological tests. More rapid and more accurate performance was seen in the Stroop interference and Trails A and B test. Both of these tests involve a condition in which a competing response tendency has to be suppressed while attention is focussed on the relevant stimulus dimension. This is usually associated with a marked slowing of performance over the non-competing control condition. The slowing effect was highly significantly attenuated in the tryptophan depleted subjects. They perform more quickly and more accurately. When they were asked to tap the space bar on a keyboard, the tryptophan depleted group tapped twice as fast. These results are analogous to the effects of 5-HT depletion in animals noted earlier. It will be interesting to determine whether reward-induced activations of dopaminergic systems using fMRI or PET will be greater after tryptophan depletion.

We have used fMRI to image the forebrain regions concerned behavioural inhibition and show that 5-HT enhances functioning in these areas [32]. This involved a GO-NO/GO paradigm in which subjects were required to press a button every time they saw an alphabetic letter unless it was the letter V in which case they were required to withhold the button press. The stimuli occurred quite rapidly so that successful response inhibition required significant attention. The regional BOLD signal in the GO condition was subtracted from the NO/GO condition to reveal regions of the brain active in association with behavioural inhibition. In keeping with a number of other studies, a focus of activation was seen in the right ventral lateral frontal cortex. Interestingly, this is close to a region which was activated when subjects viewed an angry face rather than a neutral face [33]. The perception of anger in others' faces is a powerful inhibitory social signal for humans. Elliott and Frith have summarised various imaging studies in humans which suggest that ventro-lateral frontal cortex may be part of a final common pathway of behavioural inhibition triggered by various environmental cues [34].

We repeated the experiment in the same subjects after an intravenous infusion of a drug which stimulates 5-HT2 receptors, mCPP [35]. There was a significant enhancement of the ventro-lateral frontal focus associated with behavioural inhibition. This suggests that 5-HT facilitates ventral frontal mechanisms concerned with behavioural inhibition. Interestingly, this area has a high concentration of 5-HT uptake sites and reduced concentrations have been found in post-mortem brains of suicides [36]. This has been associated with the impulsive component of suicide or suicidal behaviour. It can be seen that impaired 5-HT function could be associated with impulsive behaviour through secondary impairment of frontal behavioural inhibitory mechanisms.

Is 5-HT function abnormal in impulsive personality disordered subjects?

A number of studies have reported low concentrations of the 5-HT metabolite 5HIAA in cerebral spinal fluid in association with impulsive/aggressive personality traits. Three studies by the same group [37, 38, 39] report that violent or impulsive alcoholic offenders have significantly lower levels than non-impulsive and controls. Brown et al. [40] reported that patients in the US Navy scores of lifetime aggression had low csf 5HIAA concentrations. Lidburg et al. [41] found that impulsive suicide attemptives had lower csf 5HIAA levels than controls although concentration in murderers were no different. There has been a long debate about whether 5HIAA levels in lumbar csf reflects brain 5-HT turnover and release.

5-HT2 drug challenge studies provide a more dynamic index in brain 5-HT function than csf metabolites. Fenfluramine releases 5-HT and the resulting stimulation of 5-HT2 receptors in the hypothalamus causes the pituitary secretion of prolactin. A number of studies report attenuated prolactin responses to fenfluramine in impulsive personality disordered populations [42, 43, 44]. In Manchester, Dolan et al. reported that psychopathic murderers had attenuated responses compared to a control sample and that this correlated inversely with various questionnaire measures of impulsivity [42, 43]. The directly acting 5-HT2C receptor agonist, mCPP also evokes prolactin responses and cortisol responses. Handelsman et al. found that prolactin responses inversely correlated with the personality dimensions of hostility and depression in a population of recently detoxified alcoholics [45]. In contrast, the opposite relationship was found in recently detoxified cocaine addicts [46]. Wetzler et al. found no association between prolactin responses to mCPP and measures of aggression in a mixture of patients with depression, panic disorder and suicidal attempts [47].

We have attempted to develop a drug challenge in which the brain's response is directly visualised using fMRI [35]. An eight minute baseline scan was carried out while subjects performed visual analogue ratings of anxiety, light-headedness, uncomfortable and other subjective ratings. IV mCPP 0.08 mg/kg or placebo was administered followed by a repeat eight-minute scan with visual analogue ratings. A number of regions were activated, all of which are known to have a high concentration of 5-HT2C receptors. Most strikingly the hypothalamus was activated and the magnitude of this activation correlated with the prolactin response measured over the following 60 minutes. mCPP also increases body temperature and induces anorexia and these can be seen as hypothalamic functions. Other areas included anterior cingulate, ventral striatum, amygdala and substantia nigra. We are currently investigating the magnitude of the mCPP response in patients with impulsive personality disorders and comparing not only with controls, but also, in patients with generalised anxiety disorder who may in some regards lie at the opposite end of an anxiety behavioural inhibition continual from impulsive patients.

Antisocial personality disorder: a disorder of the anterior 5-HT-behavioural restraint system

In summary, the following lines of evidence suggest that antisocial personality disorder may indeed be a 5-HT-deficiency disorder but specifically of the anterior 5-HT behavioural restraint system:

- 5-HT opposes the effect of dopamine on incentive motivation and the behavioural response to stimulant drugs
- decreased 5-HT function in animals is associated with sensitised dopaminergic function and there is indirect evidence of this in humans
- this offers a plausible mechanism for the association between impulsive personality disorder and drug abuse in antisocial individuals
- 5-HT facilitates frontal lobe inhibitory control
- there is evidence of impaired 5-HT neurotransmitter function in murderers

It can be seen that much of the evidence is still indirect. At the least, impaired 5-HT functioning is a candidate mechanism for impulsive behaviour and addiction.

Depression and the posterior 5HT — resilience system

Normal functions of the posterior 5HT-resilience system

Like impulsive personality disorder, depression has also been associated with 5-HT deficiency. The suggestion here is that the 5-HT deficiency affects a different forebrain 5-HT system from the anterior system of behavioural inhibition. As noted earlier, the posterior group of 5-HT cells in the median raphe nucleus principally innervate the hippocampus and restricted areas of limbic cortex. Animal behavioural studies suggest that this system is concerned with adaptation to aversion. For example, Petrie et al. placed rats on a small platform some height off the ground. This produced signs of fear such as defaecation and urination but the animals became habituated when the experience was repeated every day [48]. They showed that daily exposure to the elevated platform was associated with a progressive increase in 5HT release in the hippocampus. That the increased 5HT release mediated the behavioural adaptation is suggested by studies in which intra-hippocampal injections of 5HT agonists after a single stress, prevented the expression of fear-like behaviour 24hrs later [49]. I proposed with Graeff that the human corollary is that the posterior 5HT system operates as a resilience mechanism which allows normal behaviour to resume in the face of chronic psychosocial adversity [16]. Depression occurs if the 5HT resilience coping mechanism fails. I will discuss the nature of resilience later.

Is 5-HT function abnormal in depression?

Many studies have reported reduced 5HIAA concentration in csf taken from depressed subjects. However, a surprising number have found no difference [50]. More consistent evidence for abnormal 5-HT function has come from the neuroendocrine strategy. In particular, many studies report attenuated responses following intravenous administration of the 5-HT precursor, tryptophan [4, 51]. Experiments with antagonists suggests that that growth hormone and prolactin responses to tryptophan are mediated by the 5-HT1A receptor, thought to be located in the hypothalamus [51]. It seems significant that the 5-HT1A receptor is preferentially localised in hippocampus, the terminal field of posterior raphe 5-HT cells.

As noted above, fenfluramine evoked hormonal responses are thought to be mediated by the 5-HT2C receptor. While it is often claimed that hormonal responses to fenfluramine are attenuated in depression, the evidence is in fact not clear. In general, blunting has only been observed in post-hoc comparisons in sub-groups of depressed patients — in one study in an endogenously depressed subgroup [52] and in another, non-endogenously depressed [53]. Larger studies find no differences [54].

We carried out one of the largest studies involving about 148 placebo-controlled fenfluramine challenges [55]. The study was carried out in out-patients. Overall we observed increases in prolactin responses in the depressives. We suggested that this might be a reflection of over-activity in anterior raphe anticipatory anxiety mechanisms. Interestingly, the increase was only seen if depressed patients had experienced a life-event. Depressed patients with no experience of a life-event in fact had lower prolactin responses. The results suggested to us the possibility that depression involves a pre-synaptic deficit of 5-HT release which in hippocampus and other terminal areas of the posterior raphe 5-HT system, would give rise to depressed mood and cognitions. This would be mediated by reduced activation of post-synaptic 5-HT1A receptors. In the terminal fields of the anterior raphe, aversive cues and stressors would evoke a small amount of 5-HT release playing onto super-sensitive 5-HT2 receptors giving rise to exaggerated 5-HT2 neurotransmission and symptoms of anticipatory anxiety and fear.

Stress hormones and depression

It is widely held that stress hormones have some part to play in the generation of depression, perhaps by interfering with 5-HT neurotransmission. In our recent study of 500 women in the community, morning and evening salivary cortisols were not increased in the 98 cases of depression we found, compared to the 348 controls [55]. However, the method was able to detect an effect of life-events in the last month — 50 subjects with a recent severe life-event had increased cortisol secretion. We concluded that common depression in the community while certainly associated with acute and chronic social adversity was not associated with high levels of cortisol.

Measures of chronic stress had no overall effect on plasma cortisol but within the depressed sub-group, cortisol levels were significantly greater in those with chronic psychosocial stressors than in those without. There was no effect of chronic stress on cortisol in the large number of non-depressed subjects. This result suggests that depression or its underlying vulnerability causes abnormal cortisol responses to stress. In other words, a cortisol response to chronic psychosocial stress is a manifestation of depression and not a cause. This result is reminiscent of the fenfluramine responses noted earlier; life-events affected 5-HT function only in the depressed population. No effect was seen in the non-depressed group. The results suggest that the biological mechanisms of depression involve dysregulation of 5-HT and HPA responses to acute and chronic stressors. The ability to mount a 5-HT response to chronic adversity may be an important protective mechanism in depression.

The nature of resilience

As noted earlier, Guimaraes and colleagues [49] showed that microinjections into the hippocampus of drugs increasing 5HT function (imipramine, zimelidine and the 5-HT1A agonist, N,N-dimethyltryptamine) prevented the effect of restraint stress on subsequent anxiety. Injection of glutamate antagonists also abolished the anxiogenic effect 24 hours later [56]. No effect of drug administration was seen if the injections into the hippocampus occurred before the immobilisation stress or were delayed for more than six hours after it or if they were injected immediately prior to the testing on the plus maze. These experiments are formally analogous to studies of memory consolidation in the experimental animal. Many studies have shown that amnesic agents only impair long-term retention of learned behaviours if administration occurs immediately after acquisition in the post-training period. Deakin and Graeff [16] suggested that one function of 5-HT release in hippocampus is to interfere with memory for aversive events so that they do not intrude into consciousness or continue to influence behaviour. When this 5-HT1A mediated effect breaks down, depression would be the result.

Depression clearly involves excessive rumination and attention to current and previous aversive events. Each rehearsal enhances consolidation. It is thought the hippocampus may have a role in distributing memory throughout the neo-cortex. This may be the process by which episodic memories eventually become knowledge and beliefs. In depression, repeated rehearsal and reoccurrences of aversive episodes become depressive beliefs about the self and future played out to a distributed representation in neocortex by the hippocampus. Depressive beliefs about the self and future influence the cortical processing & interpretation of future experiences and future plans. Patients define themselves by these beliefs. Hippocampal 5HT may function to prevent the transition from aversive memories to depressive beliefs/knowledge about the self and future. Depression may also involve an excessive intrusion into conscious awareness of aversive memories. Abnormalities of autobiographical memory have been described in patients with depression who show an enhanced ability to recall negative memories and an impaired ability to record pleasurable ones [57]. Hippocampal 5-HT release during aversive events may serve to limit rehearsal of aversive memories and allow normal behaviour to emerge. This maybe one mechanism of resilience.

Imaging the 5HT resilience system in depression

A recent PET imaging study suggests that these speculations based largely on animal behavioural studies maybe true in humans. Mayberg et al. [58] carried out fluorodeoxyglucose PET scans to measure regional brain metabolic activity before and after four weeks treatment with fluoxetine in patients with depression. They observed increased metabolism in a brainstem region which would appear to correspond very closely to the median raphe nucleus. In addition, they showed that metabolism decreased bilaterally in the hippocampal formation. These findings are remarkably compatible with the proposal that median raphe hippocampal 5-HT function is impaired in depression and that antidepressant drugs work by restoring function in this system.

Conclusion

— Studies in humans suggest impairment of 5-HT in neurotransmission occurs both in depression and impulse control disorders
— Different 5-HT systems mediate adaptive responses to future and current adversity
— 5HT cells in the anterior raphe modulate dopamine function and prevent contact with future threats
— Impaired 5-HT restraint of behaviour and of dopamine function is a plausible mechanism of impulsivity and addiction
— 5HT cells in the posterior raphe innervate hippocampus and limbic cortex to reduce processing of current and past aversive events in awareness and memory
— Impaired 5-HT modulation of memory is one mechanism of depression

References

1. Linnoila VM, Virkkunen M (1992) Aggression, suicidality and serotonin. low 5HT syndrome. J Clin Psychiatry 53 [Suppl 1]: 46–51
2. Delgado PL (2000) Depression: the case for a monoamine deficiency. J Clin Psychiatry 61 [Suppl 6]: 7–11
3. Newman ME, Shapira B, Lerer B (1998) Evaluation of central serotonergic function in affective and related disorders by the fenfluramine challenge test: a critical review. Int J Neuropsychopharmacol 1(1): 49–69
4. Deakin JFW, Pennell I, Upadhyaya AK, Lofthouse R (1990) A neuroendocrine study of 5HT function in depression: evidence for biological mechanisms of endogenous and psychosocial causation. Psychopharmacol 101: 85–92
5. Kapfhammer HP, Hippius H (1998) Special feature: pharmacotherapy in personality disorders. J Personal Disord 12(3): 277–288
6. Whitaker-Azmitia PM (1999) The discovery of serotonin and its role in neuroscience. Neuropsychopharmacol 21 [Suppl 2]: 2S–8S
7. Amin AH, Crawford TBB, Gaddum JH (1954) The distribution of substance P and 5-hydroxytryptamine in the central nervous system of the dog. J Physiol 126: 596–618
8. Dahlstrom A, Fuxe K (1964) Evidence for the existence of monoamine-containing neurons in the central nervous system. Acta Physiol Scand 62: 5–55
9. Baker KG, Halliday GM, Tork I (1990) Cytoarchitecture of the human dorsal raphe nucleus. J Comp Neurol 301: 147–161
10. Morris JS, Smith KA, Cowen PJ, Friston KJ, Dolan RJ (1999) Covariation of activity in habenula and dorsal raphe nuclei following tryptophan depletion. Neuro Image 10: 163–172
11. Deakin JFW (1996) 5HT, antidepressant drugs and the psychosocial origins of depression. J Psychopharmacol 10(1): 31–38
12. Imai H, Steindler DA, Kitai ST (1986) The organization of divergent axonal projections from the midbrain raphe nuclei in the rat. J Comp Neurol 243: 363–380

13. Vertes RP (1991) A PHA-L analysis of ascending projections of the dorsal raphe nucleus in the rat. J Comp Neurol 313: 643–668
14. Vertes RP, Fortin WJ, Crane AM (1999) Projections of the median raphe nucleus in the rat. J Comp Neurol 407: 555–582
15. Deakin JFW (1983) Roles of serotonergic systems in escape, avoidance and other behaviours. In: Cooper JS (ed) Theory in psychopharmacology. Academic Press, New York, pp 149–193
16. Deakin JFW, Graeff FG (1991) 5-HT and mechanisms of defence. J Psychopharmacol 5: 305–315
17. Olds J, Milner P (1954) Positive reinforcement produced by electrical stimulation of the septal area and other regions of the rat brain. J Comp Physiol Psychiatry 47: 419–427
18. Garris PA, Kilpatrick M, Bunin MA, Michael D, Walker QD, Wightman RM (1999) Dissociation of dopamine release in the nucleus accumbens from intracranial self-stimulation. Nature 398(6722): 67–69
19. Hyman SE, Malenka RC (2001) Addiction and the brain: the neurobiology of compulsion and its persistence. Nature Rev Neurosci 2: 695–703
20. Elliott R, Friston KJ, Dolan RJ (2000) Dissociable neural responses in human reward systems. J Neurosci 20(16): 6159–6165
21. Koepp MJ, Gunn RN, Lawrence AD, Cunningham VJ, Dagher A, Jones T, Brooks DJ, Bench CH, Grasby PM (1998) Evidence for striatal dopamine release during a video game. Nature 393(6682): 266–268
22. Fulford AJ, Marsden CA (1998) Conditioned release of 5-hydroxytryptamine in vivo in the nucleus accumbens following isolation-rearing in the rat. Neuroscience 83: 481–487
23. Jacobs BL, Fornal CA (1991) Activity of brain serotonergic neurons in the behaving animal. Pharmacol Rev 43: 563–578
24. Schulz W, Dayan P, Montague PR (1998) A neural substrate of prediction and reward. Science 275: 1593–1599
25. Tye NC, Iversen SD (1975) Some behavioural signs of morphine withdrawal blocked by condition stimuli. Nature 255(5507): 416–418
26. Sommer W, Möller C, Wiklund L, Thorsell A, Rimondini R, Nissbrandt H, Heilig M (2001) Local 5,7-dihydroxytryptamine lesions of rat amygdala: release of punished drinking, unaffected plus-maze behavior and ethanol consumption. Neuropsychopharmacol 24: 430–440
27. Robbins TW (1997) Arousal systems and attentional processes. Biol Psychol 45: 57–71.
28. Harrison AA, Everitt BJ, Robbins TW (1997) Doubly dissociable effects of median- and dorsal-raphe lesions on the performance of the five-choice serial reaction time test of attention in rats. Behav Brain Res 89(1–2): 135–149
29. Fletcher PJ, Korth KM, Chambers JW (1999) Selective destruction of brain serotonin neurons by 5,7-dihydroxytryptamine increases responding for a conditioned reward. Psychopharmacol (Berl) 147(3): 291–299
30. Rocha BA, Scearce-Levie K, Lucas JJ, Hiroi N, Castonon N, Crabbe JC, Nestlerk EJ, Hen R (1998) Increased vulnerability to cocaine in mice lacking the serotonin 1B receptor. Nature 393: 175–178
31. Deakin JFW, Anderson IM, Connell J, Mortimore C (unpublished) Effects of ATD on anxiety and cognitive measures in normal volunteers (unpublished manuscript)
32. Horn NR, Dolan M, Elliott R, Deakin JFW, Woodruff PWR (2003) Response inhibition and impulsivity: an fMRI study. Neuropsychologia (in press)
33. Blair RJ, Morris JS, Fritch CD, Perrett DI, Dolan RJ (1999) Dissociable neural responses to facial expression of sadness and anger. Brain 122(5): 883–893
34. Elliott R, Dolan RJ, Frith CD (2000) Dissociable functions in the medial and lateral orbitofrontal cortex: evidence from human neuroimaging studies. Cereb Cortex 10(3): 308–317

35. Anderson IM, Clark L, Elliott R, Kulkarni B, Williams SR, Deakin JFW (2002) 5HT2C receptor activation by m-chlorophenylpiperazine detected in humans with fMRI. Neuro Report 13(12): 1547–1551
36. Mann JJ, Huang Y, Underwood MD, Kassir SA, Oppenheim S, Kelly TM, Dwork AJ, Arango V (2000) A serotonin transporter gene promoter polymorphism (5-HTTLPR) and prefrontal cortical binding in major depression and suicide. Arch Gen Psychiatry 57(8): 729–738
37. Linnoila M, Virkkunen M, Scheinin M, Nuutila A, Rimon R, Goodwin FK (1983) Low cerebrospinal fluid 5-hydroxyindoleacetic acid concentration differentiates impulsive from nonimpulsive violent behaviour. Life Sci 33: 2609–2614
38. Virkkunen M, Nuutila A, Goodwin FK, Linnoila M (1987) CSF monoamine metabolites in male arsonists. Arch Gen Psychiatry 44: 241–247
39. Virkkunen M, Rawlings R, Tokola R, Poland RE, Guidotti A, Nemeroff CB, Bissette G, Kalogeras K, Karonen S-L, Linnoila M (1994) CSF biochemistries, glucose metabolism, and diurnal activity rhythms in alcoholic, violent offenders, fire setters, and healthy volunteers. Arch Gen Psychiatry 51: 20–27
40. Brown GI, Goodwin FK, Ballenger JC, Goyer PF, Major LF (1979) Aggression in humans correlates with cerebrospinal fluid metabolites. Psychiatry Res 1: 131–139
41. Lidberg L, Tuck JR, Asberg M, Scalia-Tomba GP, Bertilsson L (1985) Homicide, suicide and CSF 5-HIAA. Acta Psychiatr Scand 71(3): 230–236
42. Coccaro EF, Kavoussi RJ, Berman ME, Hauger RL (1996) Relationship of prolactin response to d-fenfluramine to behavioural and questionnaire assessments of aggression in personality disordered males. Biol Psychiatry 40: 157–164
43. O'Keane V, Moloney E, O'Neill H, O'Connor A, Smith C, Dinan TG (1992) Blunted prolactin responses to d-fenfluramine in sociopathy. Evidence for subsensitivity of central serotonergic function. Br J Psychiatry 160: 643–646
44. Dolan M, Deakin JFW, Roberts N, Anderson IM (2002) Serotonergic and cognitive impairment in impulsive aggressive personality disordered offenders: are there implications for treatment? Psychol Med 32(1): 105–117
45. Handelsman L, Holloway K, Kahn RS, Sturiano C, Rinaldi PJ, Bernstein DP, Siever L, Gabriel S, Cooper TB (1996) Hostility is associated with a low prolactin response to meta-chlorophenylpiperazine in abstinent alcoholics. Alcohol Clin Exp Res 20(5): 824–829
46. Handelsman L, Kahn RS, Sturiano C, Rinaldi PJ, Gabriel S, Schmeidler JP, Bernstein DP, Siever L, Cooper TB (1998) Hostility is associated with a heightened prolactin response to meta-chlorophenylpiperazine in abstinent cocaine addicts. Psychiatry Res 80(1): 1–12
47. Wetzler S, Kahn RS, Asnis GM, Korn M, van Praag HM (1991) Serotonin receptor sensitivity and aggression. Psychiatry Res 37(3): 271–279
48. Petrie RXA, Balfour DJK, Stewart CA, Reid IC (1998) The influence of chronic stress on 5-HT and 5-HTIAA release from rat dorsal hippocampus. Stanley Foundation European Bipolar Symposium, London
49. Netto SM, Guimaraes FS (1996) Role of hippocampal 5-HT1A receptors on elevated plus maze exploration after a single restraint experience. Behav Brain Res 77(1–2): 215–218
50. Lester D (1995) The concentration of neurotransmitter metabolites in the cerebrospinal fluid of suicidal individuals: a meta-analysis. Pharmacopsychiatry 28: 77–79
51. Cowen PJ (1996) Advances in psychopharmacology: mood disorders and dementia. Br Med Bull 52(3): 539–555
52. Mitchell P, Smythe G (1990) Hormonal responses to fenfluramine in depressed and control subjects. J Affect Disord 19: 43–51
53. Coccaro EF, Siever LJ, Klar HM, Maurer G, Cochrane K, Cooper TB, Mohrs RC, Davis KL (1989) Serotonergic studies in patients with affective and personality disorders; correlates with suicidal and impulsive aggressive behaviour. Arch Gen Psychiatry 46: 587–599

54. Park SB, Williamson DJ, Cowen PJ (1996) 5HT neuroendocrine function in major depression: prolactin and cortisol responses to d-fenfluramine. Psychol Med 26: 1191–1196
55. Strickland PL, Deakin JFW, Percival C, Dixon J, Gater RA, Goldberg PG (2002) Biosocial origins of depression in the community. Interactions between social adversity, cortisol and serotonin neurotransmission. Br J Psychiatry 180(2): 168–173
56. Padovan CM, Del Bel EA, Guimaraes FS (2000) Behavioral effects in the elevated plus maze of an NMDA antagonist injected into the dorsal hippocampus: influence on restraint stress. Pharmacol Biochem Behav 67(2): 325–330
57. Watkins E, Teasdale JD (2001) Rumination and overgeneral memory in depression: effects of self-focus and analytic thinking. J Abnorm Psychol 110(2): 353–357
58. Mayberg HS, Brannan SK, Tekell JL, Silva JA, Mahurin RK, McGinnis S, Jerabek PA (2000) Regional metabolic effects of fluoxetine in major depression: serial changes and relationship to clinical response. Biol Psychiatry 48: 830–843

Author's address: Prof. Dr. J. F. W. Deakin, Neuroscience and Psychiatry Unit, University of Manchester, G. 907 Stopford Bldg., Oxford Read, Manchester M13 9PT, United Kingdom, e-mail: bev.haggis@man.ac.uk

J Neural Transm (2003) [Suppl] 64: 95–103

Future directions in substance dependence research

D. Nutt, A. Lingford-Hughes and **M. Daglish**

Psychopharmacology Unit, University of Bristol, Bristol, United Kingdom

Summary. Substance dependence is a major health problem but increasing understanding of its neurobiology is likely to lead to improved prevention and treatment. Fundamental aspects of dependence include tolerance and withdrawal and the fact that the drug becomes the centre of the addict's world. Neuroimaging has been key in defining underlying neurobiological mechanisms. The activity in particular brain regions has been shown to be altered in addiction. These include the anterior cingulate which is involved in emotional salience and the orbitofrontal cortex, involved in impulse control. Dopamine is the key neurotransmitter since most abused drugs increase its levels, and many pharmacotherapies have targeted this system. The opiate system is also key in mediating the pleasurable effects of some drugs such as alcohol by increasing dopamine levels. The GABA and glutamate systems mediate many of the other effects of alcohol. As the neurobiology of different components of addiction become evident, pharmacological approaches involve exploiting our new understanding which will likely lead to improved treatments.

Introduction

Substance dependence (including alcohol and tobacco) is one of the major health problems in the present world with huge social as well as personal costs. Improving the healthcare aspects of substance abuse requires better understanding of the brain mechanisms of the different elements of substance dependence including tolerance, dependence and addiction (Table 1). Tolerance is the process whereby drug use leads to loss of effect with the need for larger doses to be taken in order to maintain effect. Tolerance is a feature of most drug dependence and although it may not be as apparent with the psychedelic types of drugs; this may help explain why these drugs seem to lead to less addiction. Dependence is a common consequence of tolerance and is defined loosely as loss of control and problems trying to stop using the drug. Physical withdrawal symptoms are generally present, though less so with stimulants, but there is often also a psychological element to the experience. Addiction is in a way the extreme end of this spectrum and is best conceptualised as a state of dependence in which there is also significant craving for the drug to the extent that it disrupts the individual's life. The drug

Table 1. Key concepts in substance dependence

• tolerance	= loss of efficacy
• dependence	= loss of control & problems stopping – physical +/– psychological
• addiction	= both of the above + desire/craving – lifestyle centres on drug (salience) – often loss of job, family etc.

becomes the centre of attention for the user to a degree that it takes over from other more usual sources of pleasure and reward such as family and work. In the extreme, but sadly too common, case eventually the drug so dominates the user's life that all other interests are lost and they turn to crime or self damaging behaviours such as prostitution to finance their habit (Table 1).

Intervening in the early stages of this process whereby use leads to tolerance and dependence may have some value in reducing dependence as there is some evidence that the initial use of drugs is for pleasure but during the course of a substance misuse career avoidance of the consequences of dependence especially withdrawal symptoms takes priority.

The brain circuits of substance dependence

Understanding the processes underlying these conditions requires a multidisciplinary approach, which is basically from one of two main directions for this field. The first comes from work to define the brain circuits of drug action and addiction, based on the premise that such knowledge may lead to an integration of approaches from the different elements of modern neuropsychiatry. Understanding systems may also lead to more targeted treatments such as are emerging from the study of the GABA-A receptor subtypes as discussed below. The second is to examine the neurochemical bases of addiction.

Neuroimaging, using both radionuclides (PET and SPECT) and fMRI, is being used to explore the brain circuits of addiction. This is being done from two directions. The first is to understand the sites at which drugs of dependence work in the brain and the second is to plot the brain circuits underlying different elements of addiction such as withdrawal, rush, craving and urge to use.

Some of the first studies in this area were rather counter-intuitive as they found quite profound global reductions in brain metabolism with administration of both opioids and stimulants. Work in pain patients using ^{15}O-water PET activation found that the analgesic actions of opioids were mediated by or associated with changes in brain metabolism in the anterior cingulate gyrus (Jones et al., 1991). More recently in an elegant SPECT study Schlaepfer et al. (1998) found that the reinforcing (pleasurable) actions of the mu opiate receptor agonist morphine were associated with activation in a number of brain regions including a large activation of the anterior cingulate cortex. In contrast, the kappa receptor agonist/antagonist butorphanol, which is not reinforcing but rather produces dysphoria did not activate this circuit producing marked temporal lobe changes instead.

Over the same period there have been a series of parallel studies trying to define the brain circuits underlying the different processes of addiction such as craving, pleasure, and withdrawal. These tend to use psychological provocation (e.g. Childress et al., 1999; Wang et al., 1999) of these states in the scanner although one or two studies have precipitated withdrawal pharmacologically (e.g. Van Dyck et al., 1994). Typically subjects are exposed to memories of drug craving, or use, by means of video or audio presentations of drug related paraphernalia or personal experiences. Scanning then explores changes in the metabolism or blood flow using a neutral or other stimulus exposure as the control condition. Studies in this way have looked at the brain regions involved in cocaine and opiate craving using both PET (Grant et al., 1996; Childress et al., 1999; Daglish et al., 2001) and fMRI (Maas et al., 1998) with studies of alcohol craving in their infancy. Taken together several themes emerge. The anterior cingulate cortex is implicated (activated) in most of these paradigms, but is also activated by other stimuli of emotional salience to humans such as sexual images. It therefore appears that this brain region is involved in detecting and perhaps assessing the emotional valence to and memories of drug use.

In contrast another frontal cortex region, the orbitofrontal cortex, seems more involved in the processes relating to the use of drug. Studies by several groups (London et al., 2000; Volkow and Fowler, 2000) have demonstrated associations between orbitofrontal cortex activation and cocaine use, and our own study in heroin addicts found that activation in this region correlated with the urge to use heroin (Daglish et al., 2001). We are currently using analysis techniques to examine neural connectivity to explore which other brain regions may link with the orbitofrontal cortex in producing this effect (Daglish et al., in preparation). An interesting aspect of these findings is that they share similarities with other psychiatric disorders, in particular obsessive compulsive disorder (OCD). There is an extensive body of literature that finds overactivity of cortical-subcortical loops in OCD, especially involving the orbitofrontal cortex — basal ganglia circuit (Baxter et al., 1987, see review by Malizia, 2002).

This parallelism between the neurobiology of OCD and addiction has face validity as addicts experience huge compulsions to use drugs just as OCD patients have powerful compulsions to conduct rituals. Although in OCD there is almost always resistance to these urges, this too is seen in a large proportion of addicts. Damage to the orbitofrontal cortex can lead to impulsive behaviour such as seen in many addicts and may be caused by the neurotoxic effects of the drugs themselves as stimulants may damage the 5-HT inputs to this brain region (Rogers et al., 1999).

One interesting potential benefit of this commonality between addiction and OCD in terms of brain circuits is this intriguing possibility that treatments effective in one may work in the other. The SSRIs are the mainstay of OCD therapy achieving partial remission in the majority of patients however their use in treating addicts has been mixed but adequate trials are lacking. Baxter's group and others have shown that effective treatment of OCD either by drugs or behaviour therapy rectifies the overactive brain circuit (Baxter et al., 1992; Azari et al., 1993; Brody et al., 1997).

Neurotransmitters and substance dependence

The second growth area relates to the biological underpinning of addiction in terms of neurotransmitters and hormones. This area has developed rapidly in recent years due to two factors. The first is the discovery of the role of various neurotransmitter systems being affected by the drugs of addiction and the use of genetic manipulations in animals to define genotypes that might confer vulnerability and resistance to becoming dependent on drugs.

Dopamine

The neurotransmitter that has had most focus in the past decade is dopamine as, in animal microdialysis studies, most abused drugs increase dopamine in striatal areas especially the ventral striatum or nucleus accumbens (Koob and Le Moal, 2001). In humans, PET and SPECT studies have found that several stimulants (cocaine, amphetamine and methylphenidate) release dopamine (Volkow et al., 1997, 2001). We are currently extending these studies to see if dopamine release is important in the actions of heroin. However many other stimuli both pleasurable (food, sex) and unpleasant (pain) also release dopamine in this region and dopamine release is now conceptualised to relate to anticipation, the salience of the experience, or stimuli predicting the experience, rather than drug pleasure per se (Schultz, 2001).

Nevertheless there is evidence that manipulating dopamine release may be an interesting way to develop new treatment approaches. Cocaine acts to a large extent through blocking the dopamine uptake site (Koob and Le Moal, 2001) and early studies with a selective dopamine uptake blocker GBR12909 revealed that it could reduce the actions of cocaine in animals presumably by blocking access of cocaine to the active site on the transporter (Rothman et al., 1991). For reasons not yet clear clinical trials of this agent have not yet been conducted or at least reported. Another approach is to partially block the actions of dopamine using a partial agonist at the D2/3 receptor, BP-897, (Pilla et al., 1999). The idea here is that when cocaine-dependent animals are be trained to work for cocaine by a cue (e.g. a light) that predicts cocaine availability, presentation of the cue leads to conditioned dopamine release in the nucleus accumbens before they get the cocaine. In fact this conditioned release may be the reason they continue to work to get the cocaine.

BP-897 is a dopamine receptor partial agonist that itself is not self-administered by rats, but it does block the actions of endogenous dopamine so reduces the rats interest in working for cocaine which eventually leads to an extinction of the cocaine responding behaviour. This may mean that BP-897 will be 'anti-craving' in man by reducing use in response to cues. It is currently in trials for the prevention of relapse to smoking and may soon be tested in other forms of addiction in which conditioned cues are a prominent cause of relapse e.g. cocaine and heroin dependence. Interestingly there is also some evidence that low levels of dopamine in nucleus accumbens is associated with or even causal of withdrawal symptoms from several drugs of abuse. BP-897 might also protect against this, by "replacing" the deficiency of endogenous dopamine without itself being addictive.

Another drug that is used in dependence and which may act through the dopamine system is bupropion. This is an antidepressant that in clinical trials of depression was found to reduce cigarette withdrawal symptoms. It has since obtained a licence for this indication in many countries under the trade name Zyban. Bupropion is thought to act as a mixed noradrenaline and dopamine uptake blocker, and improves the one year outcome in smoking cessation studies by up to 100% (i.e. from 15 to 30% achieving success)(Jorenby et al., 1999). A plausible explanation for this action is that bupropion minimises the presumed deficiency of dopamine thought to occur in nicotine withdrawal.

Opioid systems

Brain opiate receptors are involved in both the pleasurable and the unwanted actions of abused opioids as well as in the actions of many other drugs of dependence, particularly alcohol (Herz, 1997). An important advance in the therapy of opiate addiction has been the development of the partial agonist, buprenorphine. This acts as a mu receptor partial agonist and a kappa receptor antagonist. As a partial agonist it has significantly less effect on the respiratory system than full agonists such as heroin and methadone and so even in overdose it does not produce respiratory arrest (see Fig. 1 and Nutt, 1997). Its partial agonist properties also mean that users are less intoxicated ("gouched out") and report feeling more "normal" on buprenorphine than on methadone (Law et al., 1997). This may also relate to the lack of kappa mediated dysphoric effects.

GABA

There is evidence that GABA is involved in the action of alcohol and benzodiazepines and that reducing GABA-A function with, for example benzodiazepine receptor inverse agonists, can offset the actions of these drugs (see Lister and Nutt, 1987; Nutt, 1999; Nutt and Malizia, 2001). Modulating GABA-A receptor function downwards is difficult due to the risk of anxiety and seizures (Pratt et al., 1988; Kalueff and Nutt, 1997). However the discovery of the multiple subtypes of the GABA-A receptor and synthesis of drugs selective to some of these offers an interesting and novel approach. For instance it has been found that the α5-subtype receptor (which is found in high amounts in the hippocampus) may be important in the actions of alcohol (June et al., 2001). An inverse agonist at this receptor has recently been

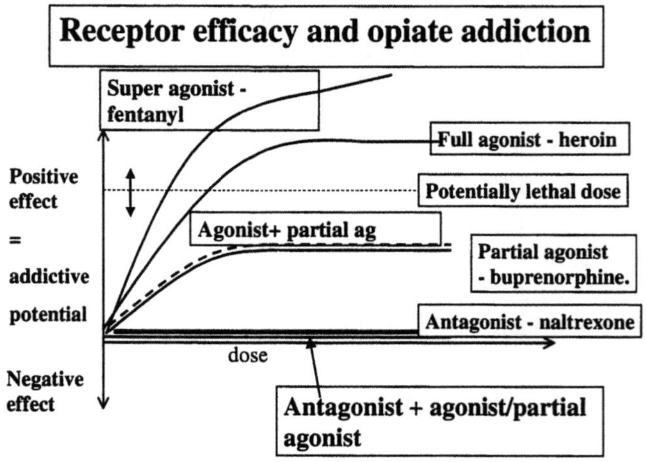

Fig. 1. Opioid efficacy at the mu opiate receptor and clinical effects

discovered (L822179) and it could be predicted that this might have anti-alcohol properties; such studies in rodents and man now need to be conducted.

Glutamate

Glutamate is the brain's principle excitatory neurotransmitter and its role in addiction is increasingly recognised. For instance, glutamatergic neurons from the prefrontal cortex (PFC) and amygdala project onto the mesolimbic reward pathway play a role in reinstatement of stimulant seeking-behaviour. The NMDA glutamate receptor has been implicated in nicotine, ethanol, benzodiazepines and cannabinoids addiction (see Wolf et al., 1998). Increased glutamatergic function underlies many features of alcohol withdrawal, including neuronal death, for which acamprosate may be protective (Dahchour and de Witte, 2000).

Substance P

There is growing interest in substance P receptors as targets for new therapeutic agents starting from the finding that a substance P antagonist was antidepressant (Kramer et al., 1998). Although the presence in the brain of substance P has been known for nearly 20 years, its role in addiction is increasingly recognised (Huston et al., 1993). This stems from several lines of evidence particularly the studies of Murtra et al. (2000) who, using substance P (NK1) receptor knockout mice, demonstrated that loss of NK1 receptors in the nucleus accumbens decreased opiate but not cocaine reward. Moreover increased substance P release has been demonstrated in ventral striatum of rats expecting to self-administer opiates, but not when expecting cocaine

(Cappendijk et al., 1999). In parallel there has been increased activity in the pharmaceutical industry and now several companies have specific and selective substance P antagonists in development. One of these has been labelled with ^{11}C as a PET ligand by the IRSL and preliminary data suggest good kinetics (Bergstrom et al., 2000).

Conclusions

Although substance dependence is one of the least-well treated areas of medicine recent research is beginning to elucidate the brain mechanisms underlying the various elements of addiction. The mode of action of most abused drugs is becoming understood and new pharmacological approaches to treatment based on receptor targets and improved kinetic profiles are being developed. These new developments are likely to lead to improved diagnosis and outcome for future generations of substance abusers.

References

Azari NP, Pietrini P, Horwitz B, Pettigrew KD, Leonard HL, Rapoport JL, Schapiro MB, Swedo SE (1993) Individual differences in cerebral metabolic patterns during pharmacotherapy in obsessive-compulsive disorder: a multiple regression/discriminant analysis of positron emission tomographic data. Biol Psychiatry 34(11): 798–809

Baxter LR Jr, Phelps ME, Mazziotta JC, Guze BH, Schwartz JM, Selin CE (1987) Local cerebral glucose metabolic rates in obsessive compulsive disorder: a comparison with rates in unipolar depression and in normal controls. Arch Gen Psychiatry 44(3): 211–218

Baxter LR Jr, Schwartz JM, Bergman KS, Szuba MP, Guze BH, Mazziotta JC, Alazraki A, Selin CE, Ferng HK, Munford P et al (1992) Caudate glucose metabolic rate changes with both drug and behavior therapy for obsessive-compulsive disorder. Arch Gen Psychiatry 49(9): 681–689

Bergstrom M, Fasth KJ, Kilpatrick G, Ward P, Cable KM, Wipperman MD, Sutherland DR, Langstrom B (2000) Brain uptake and receptor binding of two [11C]labelled selective high affinity NK1-antagonists, GR203040 and GR205171–PET studies in rhesus monkey. Neuropharmacology 39: 664–670

Brody AL, Saxena S, Schwartz JM, Stoessel PW, Maidment K, Phelps ME, Baxter LR Jr (1998) FDG-PET predictors of response to behavioral therapy versus pharmacotherapy in obsessive-compulsive disorder. Psychiatry Res: Neuroimaging 84(1): 1–6

Cappendijk SL, Hurd YL, Nylander I, van Ree JM, Terenius L (1999) A heroin-, but not a cocaine-expecting, self-administration state preferentially alters endogenous brain peptides. Eur J Pharmacol 365(2–3): 175–182

Childress AR, Mozley PD, McElgin W, Fitzgerald J, Reivich M, O'Brien CP (1999) Limbic activation during cue-induced cocaine craving. Am J Psychiatry 156(1): 11–8

Daglish MRC, Weinstein A, Malizia AL, Wilson SJ, Melichar JK, Britten S, Brewer C, Lingford-Hughes A, Myles JS, Grasby P, Nutt DJ (2001a) Regional cerebral blood flow changes elicited by craving memories in abstinent opiate-dependent individuals. Am J Psychiatry 158: 1680–1686

Dahchour A, De Witte P (2000) Ethanol and amino acids in the central nervous system: assessment of the pharmacological actions of acamprosate. Prog Neurobiol 60: 343–362

Grant S, London ED, Newlin DB, Villemagne VL, Liu X, Contoreggi C, Phillips RL, Kimes AS, Margolin A (1996) Activation of memory circuits during cue-elicited cocaine craving. Proc Natl Acad Sci 93(21): 12040–12045

Herz A (1997). Endogenous opioid systems and alcohol addiction. Psychopharmacology 129: 99–111

Huston JP, Hasenohrl RU, Boix F, Gerhardt P, Schwarting RK (1993) Sequence-specific effects of neurokinin substance P on memory, reinforcement, and brain dopamine activity. Psychopharmacology 112(2–3): 147–62 (Review)

Jones AK, Friston KJ, Qi LY, Harris M, Cunningham VJ, Jones T, Feinman C, Frackowiak RS (1991) Sites of action of morphine in the brain. Lancet 338: 825

Jorenby DE, Leischow SJ, Nides MA, et al (1999) A controlled trial of sustained-release bupropion, a nicotine patch, or both for smoking cessation. N Engl J Med 340: 685–691

June HL, Harvey SC, Foster KL, McKay PF, Cummings R, Garcia M, Mason D, Grey C, McCane S, Williams LS, Johnson TB, He X, Rock S, Cook JM (2001) GABA(A) receptors containing (alpha)5 subunits in the CA1 and CA3 hippocampal fields regulate ethanol-motivated behaviors: an extended ethanol reward circuitry. J Neurosci 21(6): 2166–2177

Kalueff AV, Nutt DJ (1997) The role of GABA in memory and anxiety. Anxiety 4(3): 100–110

Koob GF, Le Moal M (2001) Drug addiction, dysregulation of reward, and allostasis. Neuropsychopharmacology 24: 97–129

Kramer MS, Cutler N, Feighner J, Shrivastava R, Carman J, Sramek JJ, Reines SA, Liu G, Snavely D, Wyatt-Knowles E, Hale JJ, Mills SG, MacCoss M, Swain CJ, Harrison T, Hill RG, Hefti F, Scolnick EM, Cascieri MA, Chicchi GG, Sadowski S, Williams AR, Hewson L, Smith D, Rupniak NM, et al (1998) Distinct mechanism for antidepressant activity by blockade of central substance P receptors. Science 281(5383): 1640–1645

Law FD, Bailey JE, Allen DS, Melichar JK, Myles JS, Mitcheson MC, Lewis JW, Nutt DJ (1997) The feasibility of abrupt methadone-buprenorphine transfer in British opiate addicts in an out patient setting. Addic Biol 2(2): 191–200

Lister RG, Nutt DJ (1987) Is Ro 15–4513 a specific alcohol antagonist? Trends Neurosci 101: 223–225

London ED, Ernst M, Grant S, Bonson K, Weinstein A (2000) Orbitofrontal cortex and human drug abuse: functional imaging. Cerebral Cortex 10(3): 334–342

Maas LC, Lukas SE, Kaufman MJ, Weiss RD, Daniels SL, Rogers VW, Kukes, TJ, Renshaw PF (1998) Functional magnetic resonance imaging of human brain activation during cue-induced cocaine craving. Am J Psychiatry 155: 124–126

Malizia AL (2002) The neuroinaging of anxiety. In: Nutt DJ, Ballenger J (eds) Anxiety disorders. Blackwells, pp 201–228

Murtra P, Sheasby AM, Hunt SP, De Felipe C (2000) Rewarding effects of opiates are absent in mice lacking the receptor for substance P. Nature 405(6783): 180–183

Nutt DJ (1997) Receptor pharmacology of buprenorphine. Buprenorphine — a substitution agent for the treatment of opioid addiction: a UK perspective. Res Clin Forums 19(2): 9–15

Nutt DJ (1999) Alcohol and the brain: pharmacological insights for psychiatrists. Br J Psychiatry 175: 114–119

Nutt DJ, Malizia AL (2001) New insights into the role of the GABA-A benzodiazepine receptor. Br J Psychiatry 179: 390–396

Pratt JA, Laurie DJ, McCulloch J (1988) The effects of FG 7142 upon local cerebral glucose utilization suggest overlap between limbic structures important in anxiety and convulsions. Brain Res 475(2): 218–231

Pilla M, Perachon S, Sautel F, Garrido F, Mann A, Wermuth CG, Schwartz JC, Everitt BJ, Sokoloff P (1999) Selective inhibition of cocaine-seeking behaviour by a partial dopamine D3 receptor agonist. Nature 400: 371–375

Rogers RD, Everitt BJ, Baldacchino A, Blackshaw AJ, Swainson R, Wynne K, Baker NB, Hunter J, Carthy T, Booker E, London M, Deakin JF, Sahakian BJ, Robbins TW (1999) Dissociable deficits in the decision-making cognition of chronic amphetamine abusers, opiate abusers, patients with focal damage to prefrontal cortex, and tryptophan-depleted normal volunteers: evidence for monoaminergic mechanisms. Neuropsychopharmacology 20(4): 322–339

Rothman RB, Mele A, Reid AA, Akunne HC, Greig N, Thurkauf A, de Costa BR, Rice KC, Pert A (1991) GBR12909 antagonizes the ability of cocaine to elevate extracellular levels of dopamine. Pharmacol Biochem Behav 40(2): 387–397

Schlaepfer TE, Strain EC, Greenberg BD, Preston KL, Lancaster E, Bigelow GE, Barta PE, Pearlson GD (1998) Site of opioid action in the human brain: mu and kappa agonists' subjective and cerebral blood flow effects. Am J Psychiatry 155: 470–473

Schultz W (2001) Reward signaling by dopamine neurons. Neuroscience 7: 293–302

van Dyck CH, Rosen MI, Thomas HM, McMahon TJ, Wallace EA, O'Connor PG, Sullivan M, Krystal JH, Hoffer PB, Woods SW, Kosten TR (1994) SPECT regional cerebral blood flow alterations in naltrexone-precipitated withdrawal from buprenorphine. Psychiatry Res 55(4): 181–191

Volkow ND, Fowler JS (2000) Addiction, a disease of compulsion and drive: involvement of the orbitofrontal cortex. Cerebral Cortex 10(3): 318–325

Volkow ND, Wang GJ, Fischman MW, Foltin RW, Fowler JS, Abumrad NN, Vitkun S, Logan J, Gatley SJ, Pappas N, Hitzemann R, Shea CE (1997) Relationship between subjective effects of cocaine and dopamine transporter occupancy. Nature 386: 827–830

Volkow ND, Wang G, Fowler JS, Logan J, Gerasimov M, Maynard L, Ding Y, Gatley SJ, Gifford A, Franceschi D (2001) Therapeutic doses of oral methylphenidate significantly increase extracellular dopamine in the human brain. J Neurosci 15;21(2): RC121

Wang GJ, Volkow ND, Fowler JS, Cervany P, Hitzemann RJ, Pappas NR, Wong CT, Felder C (1999) Regional brain metabolic activation during craving elicited by recall of previous drug experiences. Life Sci 64(9): 775–784

Wolf ME (1998) The role of excitatory amino acids in behavioral sensitization to psychomotor stimulants. Prog Neurobiol 54: 679–720

Authors' address: Prof. D. Nutt, Psychopharmacology Unit, University of Bristol, Bristol BS8 1TD, United Kingdom, e-mail: david.j.nutt@bris.ac.uk

J Neural Transm (2003) [Suppl] 64: 105–117

New developments in the pharmacotherapy of schizophrenia

W. W. Fleischhacker

Department of Biological Psychiatry, Innsbruck University Clinics, Innsbruck, Austria

Summary. This review summarizes current key research strategies and the most prominently pursued new potential treatments for schizophrenia. First, new routes of administration for second generation antipsychotics are presented. These include rapidly dissolving tablets, drops and sirups as well as new intramuscular formulations. Newly available short acting and long acting (depot) antipsychotics complement oral antipsychotics so that the full spectrum of routes of administration is now available for second generation antipsychotics.

Next to antipsychotic polypharmacy, in which two or more antipsychotics are combined, pharmacological add-on treatments, mainly with benzodiazepines, antidepressants and mood stabilizers enjoy increasing popularity. Most of this practice is driven by personal preferences, clinical experience and marketing rather than evidence based medicine.

New pharmacological mechanisms currently utilized in advanced states of development include partial dopamine D2-receptor agonism, supplementation with glutamatergic agents, estrogen and omega-3-fatty acids. While the concept of partial D1-agonism has already led to the successful launch of a new antipsychotic, aripiprazole, the other attempts to improve therapeutic response in schizophrenia patients have so far provided equivocal results. It is argued that they may be helpful for certain subgroups or specific symptoms of schizophrenia patients. In conclusion, many exciting new pharmacological leads are currently pursued and this will very likely augment the options for treating patients with schizophrenia.

Introduction

The second half of the last century has seen tremendous advances in the care for people suffering from schizophrenia. This holds true both for pharmacological and psychosocial measures (see Fig. 1). This review will focus on pharmacotherapy.

A number of landmarks can be identified, when looking at the development of pharmacological agents to treat people with schizophrenia: the early 1950's saw the advent of neuroleptics, the first agents that were able to

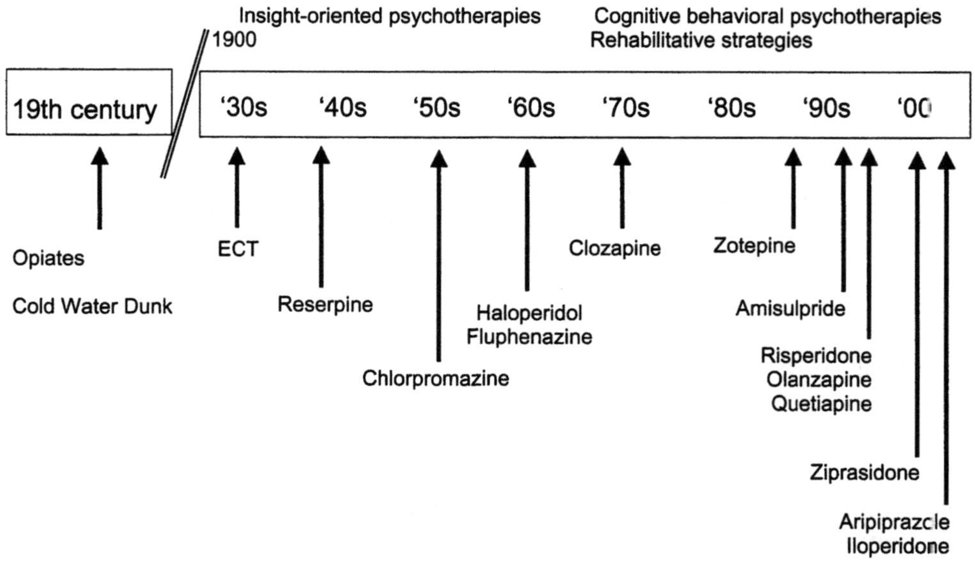

Fig. 1. Development of treatments for schizophrenia

specifically treat key symptoms of the disorder, such as hallucinations and delusions. The next two decades were characterized by the attempt to improve both the efficacy and safety of these new compounds. The introduction of long-acting injectable preparations also fell into this period. The next significant step forward was the licensing of the "anomalous" drug clozapine in Europe in the early 70's. Clozapine was the first drug that effectively treated schizophrenia symptoms without eliciting major extrapyramidal motor side effects (EPS). Although shown to be a very effective antipsychotic, its use was severely restricted by the propensity to cause agranulocytosis. Despite this, clozapine was used increasingly, and after proof was being provided that this drug is helpful for patients, who are either resistant or intolerant to other neuroleptics, clozapine was finally also approved in many countries outside of Europe. The success of clozapine also catalyzed two other advances in the field: the name antipsychotic slowly replaced the old term neuroleptic and, more importantly, researchers in the pharmaceutical industry made significant efforts to find a drug that mirrored the efficacy — but not the toxicity — of clozapine. This was done by either modifying the structure of clozapine, olanzapine being one example for this attempt, or by trying to find structurally unrelated drugs, which nevertheless shared some pharmacological properties with clozapine. Potent 5HT2 receptor antagonism is one of the examples for the latter approach, being exemplified by risperidone.

Independent of these efforts, more specific D2-antagonists, the benzamides, the latest of which is amisulpride, were brought to market.

As the main distinction of these new antipsychotics from traditional neuroleptics was their lower propensity to cause adverse motor effects, they were felt to constitute a second generation of antipsychotics (Sartorius et al., 2002). Moreover, exponentially expanding knowledge about the neurobiology of schizophrenia, seen in the context with psychopharmacological research, set the stage for drugs with new mechanisms of action so that we are currently on the threshold of a third generation of antipsychotic drugs. Partial dopamine agonists and drugs affecting glutamatergic systems are currently the most conspicuous members of this category.

Apart from these specific developments, progress has been made with regard to using the available antipsychotics more efficiently. This includes new routes of administration as well as different dosing strategies and add-on or combination treatments. Lastly, the evidence about the advantageous concomitant use of pharmacotherapy and psychosocial treatments is mounting.

New routes of administration for second generation antipsychotics

Traditional neuroleptics are available for both oral and parenteral application, the latter in the form of short acting and long acting (depot) antipsychotics. With regard to oral antipsychotics, drops and sirups complement the more conventional tablets. As the severity and quality of psychopathological symptoms differ considerably both within and between patients with schizophrenia, the preferred route of application of antipsychotic drugs varies. While acutely ill, some hostile and agitated patients may require short acting intramuscular or intravenous injections (Altamura et al., 2003). The long-term management of patients in remission or with stable symptoms is often facilitated by administration of depot injections, which maintain effective plasma levels over several weeks (Kane et al., 1998). Originally, second generation antipsychotics were only available in the oral tablet form. This, in effect, precluded their use in patients in need for alternative pharmaceutical preparations. Over the last few years, considerable progress has been made in this regard. Rapidly dissolving tablets, which are currently available for olanzapine and risperidone, were developed in order to ensure a quick resorption of the respective drugs. In addition, an acute intramuscular form is available for ziprasidone (Brook, 2000; Daniel et al., 2001), and pending for olanzapine (Wright et al., 2001). These drugs have been shown to ease the management of patients, especially in emergency psychiatry settings. A long acting preparation of risperidone (Kane et al., 2003; Eerdekens et al., 2002), embedded in dissolvable microspheres, which release the active moiety of the drug over a course of 2–3 weeks, has been launched in some countries in 2002. This means that clinicians, in principle, can now fall back on all routes of application that are and were available for the old neuroleptics, also when using second generation antipsychotics. This enhances the usefulness of the novel drugs significantly.

Pharmacological add-on treatments

Ever since neuroleptics were introduced, physicians have tried to optimize their effects by combining them with either other antipsychotics or a number of psychotropic drugs from various classes (Kiivet et al., 1995; Chong et al., 2000; Brunot et al., 2002; Rittmannsberger et al., 1999). Polypharmacy in patients with schizophrenia is probably the most popular treatment with, at the same time, the weakest justification from the available evidence.

Antipsychotic polypharmacy

The rationalizations for combining different antipsychotics are almost inexhaustible: they include the attempt to augment efficacy of one drug against positive symptoms by adding another; the wish to provide an assured base treatment with a depot antipsychotic in patients, who are felt to profit from an oral second generation antipsychotic, but have questionable compliance; the need for sedation; the perception, that patients whose positive symptoms are well controlled by traditional antipsychotics will profit from the addition of a second generation drug with respect to negative symptoms; the feeling that lower doses of two drugs induce less side effects than higher doses of a single drug, and many others. With regard to the newer antipsychotics, the curious observer is, when questioning these practices, often confronted by the fact that physicians do not really trust the efficacy of these novel agents and so, although convinced by superior safety and tolerability, feel that it is necessary to combine them with low doses of traditional antipsychotics, especially to secure control of positive symptoms. This attitude is not infrequently shared by patients and their significant others, who fear that tampering with a reasonably successful drug will put them at risk for a worsening of the disorder.

Antipsychotic polypharmacy is influenced by a host of different factors including regional preferences, subjective experience and education of clinicians, patient attitudes and perceptions, and complex interactions between patients, their relatives and the care team. It appears least influenced by data that stem from randomized controlled clinical trials. I am aware of a single placebo-controlled study that has explored adding sulpiride to clozapine in treatment-resistant patients (Shiloh et al., 1997). The addition to sulpiride was superior to placebo in this study.

In summary, it seems fair to conclude that neuroleptic polypharmacy should remain a last resort. Given the considerable amount of antipsychotics available in most countries, and the large dose ranges in which they can be used, one should first explore all possibilities of monotherapy, which may often include the need to switch patients from an unsuccessful drug to a potentially more promising antipsychotic. Adding one antipsychotic to another often just adds to the therapeutic confusion, as one can never really be sure which of the drugs that are used concomitantly is really responsible for both beneficial and adverse effects.

Antipsychotics combined with other psychotropic drugs

Antipsychotics are also combined with a host of other psychotropic agents most commonly anxiolytics, antidepressants and mood stabilizers. In contrast to the combinations discussed above, research does provide some answers for these add-on strategies.

Benzodiazepines are mainly used in three indications: agitation, concomitant anxiety and sleep disturbances, and catatonia (Wolkowitz et al., 1991; Wassef et al., 1999; Allen et al., 2001; Lingjaerde, 1991; Hawkins et al., 1995; Ungvari et al., 2001).

The sedative effects of benzodiazepines are undisputed. Clinicians take advantage of them mainly for the management of acutely agitated patients. In many instances single doses or the concomitant use of benzodiazepines for a few days suffice to resolve the problem. As benzodiazepines are safe drugs with little side effects in the short term, many clinicians prefer them over the combination of two antipsychotics. This preference is shared by patients.

Secondly, benzodiazepines can be used to counteract sleep disturbances and/or anxiety symptoms, both frequently present in schizophrenia patients. The main clinical problem in this context is the risk for abuse/dependence, when these drugs are prescribed for longer periods of time. As in the management of anxiety disorders, long-term prescriptions should be avoided and alternative strategies — both pharmacological and non-pharmacological — should be recommended. As some of the second generation antipsychotics have been shown to have better efficacy against anxiety symptoms in schizophrenia patients than their traditional counterparts (Tollefson et al., 1998; Marder et al., 1997; Müller et al., 2002), switching to these newer compounds may be indicated. Various relaxation techniques are also available to help patients cope with anxiety symptoms.

Antipsychotics combined with antidepressants

Depressive symptoms are frequent comorbid features of schizophrenia (Hausmann and Fleischhacker, 2002). A number of well controlled clinical trials have investigated the usefulness of combing antidepressants with antipsychotics (Hausmann and Fleischhacker, 2000). All evidence taken together, clinical trial data support combining these two types of drugs, although research was performed almost exclusively with tricyclic antidepressants and traditional neuroleptics. As was stated above for anxiety, some of the second generation antipsychotic drugs appear to have inbuilt antidepressant properties. Again, it would make sense to try monotherapy with these compounds first. Clinical evidence is available for amisulpride, olanzapine and risperidone (Tollefson et al., 1998; Peuskens et al., 2000, 2002), while zotepine and ziprasidone, blocking monoamine reuptake in preclinical studies (Tandon et al., 1997; Rowley et al., 1998), would also appear to be suited for this indication.

Antipsychotics combined with lithium

Lithium-antipsychotic combinations also have a long tradition in the management of schizophrenia. This applies to both the acute setting, where schizophrenia patients with elated mood are treated with this combination and maintenance and relapse prevention. More recent research of the topic does not support this practice (Schulz et al., 1999).

Antipsychotics combined with anticonvulsants

As anticonvulsants are increasingly replacing lithium salts in the treatment of affective disorders, especially in the US, this tendency has spilled over to schizophrenia patients, a large number of which now receive combinations of antipsychotics with various anticonvulsants (Clark et al., 2002; Pappadopulos et al., 2002). In contrast to lithium, such combinations have rarely been methodologically studied. A recent trial of the combination of divalproex with olanzapine or risperidone, found advantages for the combination of divalproex with either of the two drugs over monotherapy, especially with regard to onset of antipsychotic action (Casey et al., 2003b). Clearly, such findings need to be replicated. Whether or not such combinations are helpful with regard to long-term treatment remains an open question.

There is dearth of good clinical studies on the usefulness of polypharmacy, as add-on studies in schizophrenia patients are seldomly in the interest of the pharmaceutical industry (unless both components come from the same producer) and therefore unlikely to be sponsored. Psychopharmacologists convinced of the necessity of polypharmacy should therefore be encouraged to substantiate their claims and experiences by performing the relevant clinical trials.

New pharmacological mechanisms

Over the years, numerous pharmacological mechanisms, apart from the classical approach to block dopamine D2-receptors, to treat schizophrenia symptoms have been explored. Results of clinical studies have often been ambiguous and so far clinical success has not been substantial with a few notable exceptions. The following update will concentrate on those pharmacological mechanisms, which are explored clinically to date. Some experimental treatments which have provided at least partially encouraging results, such as dopamine D1-receptor antagonists against negative symptoms (Den Boer et al., 1995), specific 5HT2 antagonists against negative symptoms (Duinkerke et al., 1993), sigma antagonists against the full spectrum of the disorder (Frieboes and Steiger, 2000) and GABA-agonists (Wassef et al., 1999) will not be discussed, as, to my knowledge, these routes of intervention are currently not explored any further. In addition, mechanisms, which so far have yielded only negative results in clinical trials, for example dopamine D4-receptor antagonists (Kramer et al., 1997), will also not be covered.

Most of the interventions briefly touched upon above and outlined in more detail below, although conceived to be potential monotherapies, have so far been studied only as add-on interventions. Technically, therefore they should have been covered in the previous chapter, but since they reflect mechanisms that are clearly distinct from the traditional pharmacology of antipsychotics, they have been included into this new mechanisms section.

Partial dopamine receptor agonists

Every compound licensed to treat schizophrenia blocks dopamine D2 receptors, albeit to a varying extent. Next to the fact that it has long been recognized that shutting down dopamine receptors in all parts of the brain is responsible for a number of side effects of antipsychotics (See, 2000), more recent evidence indicates that hyperdopaminergia may only be part of the biochemical background of schizophrenia. In certain brain areas, such as the prefrontal cortex, dopamine systems are likely to be understimulated, which has been said to contribute to negative symptoms and cognitive dysfunctions (Friedman et al., 1999). If these hypotheses hold ground, an ideal antipsychotic would, firstly, block dopamine receptors in systems of increased stimulation and secondly, act as an agonist in understimulated areas. Pharmacologically, this can be accomplished by weak agonists, which can prevent a stimulation of dopamine receptors by binding to them and thereby making them unavailable for endogenous dopamine. On the other hand, these substances, being agonists, provide at least some receptor stimulation in systems, which lack the endogenous neurotransmitter. Although theoretically very appealing, a number of drugs have failed to achieve this goal, mostly because they were too strong an agonist. Examples induce pramipexole, which is now used as an antiparkinsonian drug (Benkert et al., 1995; Biglan and Holloway, 2002).

The first drug in which is this concept has succeeded in clinical studies is aripiprazole, a quinolinone derivative which is a partial agonist at dopamine D2 and serotonin 5HT1A receptors and an antagonist at 5HT2A receptors (McGavin and Goa, 2002). In a dose range of 15–30 mg per day aripiprazole monotherapy has been shown to be superior to placebo and at least as effective as haloperidol 10 mg daily (Kane et al., 2002) and risperidone 6 mg per day. Therapeutic efficacy has been shown to be maintained over the course of one year. The risk to induce extrapyramidal motor side effects appears comparable to placebo and risperidone but is significantly lower than haloperidol. Apart from the infrequent induction of EPS, aripiprazole appears to have a markedly good safety and tolerability profile, especially with regard to weight, prolactin, QTc changes and glucose and lipid metabolism (Casey et al., 2003b). Sedation was reported during the first weeks of treatment.

As all the information about this drug available to date stems from preregistration clinical trials, it needs to be supplemented by larger scale post marketing clinical studies, which are easier to generalize.

Glutamatergic agents

It has long been known that NMDA receptor antagonists such as phencylclidine (PCP) and ketamine can induce schizophrenia-like psychoses. Abberations of glutamate receptors and glutamate levels have also been revealed in post mortem studies. Many antipsychotic drugs can counteract PCP and ketamine induced deficits in various animal models for schizophrenia. As glutamatergic and dopaminergic systems are intricately linked in brain regions deemed relevant to schizophrenia, it appeared reasonable to study the effects of drugs affecting glutamatergic tone in schizophrenia patients (Goff et al., 2000).

So far, the glutamatergic agents glycine, D-cycloserine and D-serine have been studied concerning their antipsychotic efficacy (Javitt, 2002). Glycine and D-serine are full agonists at the glycine recognition site, D-cycloserine is a partial agonist. All clinical trials have been add-on studies, in which these drugs were combined with different antipsychotics, including clozapine. With the exception of the clozapine add-on studies (Evins et al., 2000; Potkin et al., 1999), all clinical trials have consistently reported a significant improvement of negative symptoms (Goff et al., 1999a; Heresco-Levy, 1999; Javitt et al., 2001) when compared to the effect of a placebo comparison group. Interestingly, there was no detectable effect on positive symptoms in any of the studies performed so far and, in some trials, cognitive deficits showed some improvement (Goff et al., 1995). When D-cycloserine was added to clozapine, none of the schizophrenia symptoms improved. D-cycloserine, when added to risperidone also led to some improvement of negative symptoms (Evins et al., 2002). AMPA receptors, a subtype of glutamatergic ionotropic receptors, have also recently become the target of therapeutic trials. Preliminary findings in about 20 patients, who were given an ampakine together with clozapine revealed an improvement in cognitive functioning compared to placebo (Goff et al., 1999b).

In summary, glutamatergic agents provide some interesting leads. They may be potentially helpful as add-on medications for the alleviation of negative symptoms or, possibly, cognitive impairment.

Omega-3-Fatty Acids

A lot of circumstantial evidence suggests that cell membrane structure may be altered in patients suffering from schizophrenia. As much of this evidence indicates that the metabolism of phospholipids and polyunsaturated fatty acids (PUFA) is abnormal in schizophrenia (Mahadik et al., 2001), a number of investigators have studied the potential therapeutic effect of PUFA supplementation. Between 1 and 4 mg of ethyl-eicosapenatenoic acid (EPA) was added to ongoing antipsychotic treatment. While a Cochrane review in the year 2000 stated that ... "results look encouraging for fish oil" (Joy et al., 2000), more recent placebo controlled clinical trials have produced equivocal evidence. The smallest study, enrolling 40 patients in South Africa (Emsley et al., 2002), reported significant advantages in symptom reduction in patients who received EPA supplementation versus placebo. A similar study, performed in the UK (Peet et al., 2001), showed superiority of EPA over placebo after 3 months, when analyzing PANSS total change scores. The same group conducted a considerably larger multicenter study which failed to find a difference between EPA augmentation and the placebo group (Peet et al., 2002). The authors attribute this to a large placebo effect. In a subgroup analysis of patients, in which EPA was added to clozapine, this combination showed a significantly better effect than clozapine plus placebo. A group of US investigators (Fenton et al., 2001) also performed a placebo-controlled study and failed to find a positive effect of EPA supplementation after 4 months with respect to residual symptoms and cognitive impairment.

In conclusion, the available evidence remains inconsistent and the field awaits further research. Maybe certain, as yet undefined, subgroups of patients, who will benefit from PUFA treatment, can be identified in future studies.

Estrogen

Epidemiological findings in the late 80's, which documented that female patients had a considerably later onset of schizophrenia than males, and clinical observations that suggested that femalè patients with high estrogen levels, as for instance during pregnancy, were less prone to suffer a psychotic relapse (Riecher-Rössler, 2002; Riecher-Rössler et al., 1994) prompted systematic investigations of the influence of female sexual hormones on psychosis. Animal studies, which demonstrated that estradiol can modulate the sensitivity of dopamine receptors in the brain (Gattaz et al., 1992) provided an additional theoretical background for the "antipsychotic" effects of estrogen. So far, a number of explorative smaller but well controlled clinical trials have been conducted (Kulkarni et al., 1996, 2002; Lindamer et al., 2001). In general, adjunctive estrogen enhanced the responsivity of symptoms, although results are somewhat inhomogenuous. As estrogen hormone replacement is not without problems in itself, the clinical merit of this strategy in schizophrenia patients remains to be discussed. Maybe its relevance will be restricted to specific patients, for instance those with estrogen deficiency syndromes.

Conclusions and future directions

This brief overview is meant to emphasize that never before have there been so many exciting and promising leads towards an improved pharmacotherapy for schizophrenia. The more we learn about the treatment of this severe psychiatric disorder, the clearer it becomes that it is unlikely that we will find a "one size fits all treatment" in the near future. The forthcoming challenge is to match specific treatments with individual patients, ideally based on biological predictors. It is not unlikely that, for instance, a postmenopausal female schizophrenia patient with low estrogen levels and severe cognitive impairment will profit most from a prolactin-sparing second generation antipsychotic combined with both estrogen replacement and a nicotinergic agonist. Exercise and a diet rich in PUFA's could also be recommended to lower cholesterol levels and enhance neural membrane synthesis. A lot of the evidence for the different pieces of this puzzle is already available, we may only need to put them together in a synthetic fashion.

References

Allen MH, Currier GW, Hughes DH, Reyes-Harde M, Docherty JP, The Expert Consensus Panel for Behavioral Emergencies (2001) The Expert Consensus Guideline Series. Treatment of behavioral emergencies. Postgrad Med: 1–88

Altamura AC, Sassella F, Santini A, Montresor C, Fumagalli S, Mun E (2003) Intramuscular preparations of antipsychotics: uses and relevance in clinical practice. Drugs 63: 493–512

Benkert O, Muller-Siecheneder F, Wetzel H (1995) Dopamine agonists in schizophrenia: a review. Eur Neuropsychopharmacol 5 [Suppl]: 43–53

Biglan KM, Holloway RG (2002) A review of pramipexole and its clinical utility in Parkinson's disease. Exp Opin Pharmacother 3: 197–210

Brook S (2000) A pilot study of intramuscular ziprasidone in the short-term treatment of patients with acute exacerbation of schizophrenia. Hum Psychopharmacol 15: 521–524

Brunot A, Lauchaux B, Sontag H, Casadebaig F, Philippe A, Rouillon F, Clery-Melin P, Hergueta T, Llorca PM, Moreaudefarges T, Guillon P, Lebrun T (2002) Pharmacoepidemiological study on antipsychotic drug prescription in French psychiatry: patients characteristics, antipsychotic treatment, and care management for schizophrenia. Encephale 28: 129–138

Casey DE, Carson WH, Saha AR, Liebeskind A, Ali MW, Jody D, Ingenito GG (2003a) Switching patients to aripiprazole from other antipsychotic agents: a multicenter randomized study. Psychopharmacology (in press)

Casey DE, Daniel DG, Wassef AA, Tracy KA, Wozniak P, Sommerville KW (2003b) Effect of divalproex combined with olanzapine or risperidone in patients with acute exacerbation of schizophrenia. Neuropsychopharmacol 28: 182–192

Chong SA, Remington GJ, Lee N, Mahendran R (2000) Contrasting clozapine prescribing patterns in the east and west? Ann Acad Med Singapore 29: 75–78

Clark RE, Bartels SJ, Mellman TA, Peacock WJ (2002) Recent trends in antipsychotic combination therapy of schizophrenia and schizoaffective disorder: implications for state mental health policy. Schizophr Bull 28: 75–84

Daniel DG, Potkin SG, Reeves KR, Swift RH, Harrigan EP (2001) Intramuscular (IM) ziprasidone 20 mg is effective in reducing acute agitation associated with psychosis: a double-blind, randomized trial. Psychopharmacology 155: 128–134

Den Boer JA, van Megen JJGM, Fleischhacker WW, Louwerens JW, Slaap BR, Westenberg HG, Burrows GD, Srivastava ON (1995) Differential effects of the D1-DA receptor antagonist SCH39166 on positive and negative symptoms of schizophrenia. Psychopharmacology 121: 317

Duinkerke SJ, Botter PA, Jansen AA, van Dongen PA, van Haaften AJ, Boom AJ, van Laarhoven JH, Busard HL (1993) Ritanserin, a selective 5-HT2/1C antagonist, and negative symptoms in schizophrenia. A placebo-controlled double blind trial. Br J Psychiatry 163: 451–455

Eerdekens M, Fleischhacker WW, Xie Y, Gefvert O (2002) Long-term safety of long-acting risperidone microspheres. Schizophr Res 53 [Suppl]: 174

Emsley R, Myburgh C, Oosthuizen P, van Rensburg SJ (2002) Randomized, placebo-controlled study of ethyl-eicosapentaenoic acid as supplemental treatment in schizophrenia. Am J Psychiatry 159: 1596–1598

Evins AE, Fitzgerald SM, Wine L, Rosselli R, Goff DC (2000) Placebo-controlled trial of glycine added to clozapine in schizophrenia. Am J Psychiatry 157: 826–828

Evins AE, Amico E, Posever TA, Toker R, Goff DC (2002) D-cycloserine added to risperidone in patients with primary negative symptoms of schizophrenia. Schizophr Res 56: 19–23

Fenton WS, Dickerson F, Boronow J, Hibbeln JR, Knable M (2001) A placebo-controlled trial of omega-3 fatty acid (ethyl eicosapentaenoic acid) supplementation for residual symptoms and cognitive impairment in schizophrenia. Am J Psychiatry 158: 2071–2074

Frieboes RM, Steiger A (2000) The antipsychotic effects of sigma drugs. In: Lidow MS (ed) Neurotransmitter receptors in actions of antipsychotic medication. CRC Press, Boca Raton London New York Washington DC, pp 137–152

Friedman JI, Temporini H, Davis KL (1999) Pharmacologic strategies for augmenting cognitive performance in schizophrenia. Biol Psychiatry 45: 1–16

Gattaz WF, Behrens S, De Vry J, Hafner H (1992) Estradiol inhibits dopamine mediated behavior in rats — an animal model of sex-specific differences in schizophrenia. Fortschr Neurol Psychiatr 60: 8–16

Goff DC (2000) Glutamate receptors in schizophrenia and antipsychotic drugs. In: Lidow MS (ed) Neurotransmitter receptors in actions of antipsychotic medication. CRC Press, Boca Raton London New York Washington DC, pp 121–136

Goff DC, Tsai G, Manoach DS, Coyle JT (1995) Dose-finding trial of D-cycloserine added to neuroleptics for negative symptoms in schizophrenia. Am J Psychiatry 152: 1213–1215

Goff DC, Tsai G, Levitt J, Amico E, Manoach D, Schoenfeld DA, Hayden DL, McCarley R, Coyle JT (1999a) A placebo-controlled trial of D-cycloserine added to conventional neuroleptics in patients with schizophrenia. Arch Gen Psychiatry 56: 21–27

Goff D et al (1999b) A preliminary dose escalation trial of CX516 (ampakine) added to clozapine in schizophrenia. Cited in: Goff DC (2000) Glutamate receptors in schizophrenia and antipsychotic drugs. In: Lidow MS (ed) Neurotransmitter receptors in actions of antipsychotic medication. CRC Press, Boca Raton London New York Washington DC, pp 121–136

Hausmann A, Fleischhacker WW (2000) Depression in patients with schizophrenia. CNS Drugs 14: 289–299

Hausmann A, Fleischhacker WW (2002) Differential diagnosis of depressed mood in patients with schizophrenia: a diagnostic algorithm based on a review. Acta Psychiatr Scand 106: 83–96

Hawkins JM, Archer KJ, Strakowski SM, Keck PE (1995) Somatic treatment of catatonia. Int J Psychiatry Med 25: 345–369

Heresco-Levy U, Javitt DC, Ermilov M, Mordel C, Silipo G, Lichtenstein M (1999) Efficacy of high-dose glycine in the treatment of enduring negative symptoms of schizophrenia. Arch Gen Psychiatry 56: 29–36

Javitt DC (2002) Glycine modulators in schizophrenia. Curr Opin Invest Drugs 3: 1067–1072

Javitt DC, Silipo G, Cienfuegos A, Shelly AM, Bark N, Park M, Lindenmayer JP, Suckow R, Zukin SR (2001) Adjunctive high-dose glycine in the treatment of schizophrenia. Int J Neuropsychopharmacol 4: 385–391

Joy CB, Mumby-Croft R, Joy LA (2000) Polyunsaturated fatty acids (fish or evening primrose oil) for schizophrenia. Cochrane Database Syst Rev: CD001257

Kane JM, Aguglia E, Altamura AC, Guitierrez JLA, Brunello N, Fleischhacker WW, Gaebel W, Gerlach J, Guelfi JD, Kissling W, Lapierre YD, Lindström E, Mendlewicz J, Racagni G, Carulla IS, Schooler NR (1998) Guidelines for depot antipsychotic treatment in schizophrenia. Eur Neuropsychopharmacol 8: 55–66

Kane JM, Carson WH, Saha AR, McQuade RD, Ingenito GG, Zimbroff DL, Ali MW (2002) Efficacy and safety of aripiprazole and haloperidol versus placebo in patients with schizophrenia and schizoaffective disorder. J Clin Psychiatry 63: 763–771

Kane JM, Eerdekens M, Lindenmayer JP, Keith SJ, Lesem M, Karcher K (2003) Long-acting injectible risperidone: efficacy and safety of the first long-acting atypical antipsychotic. Am J Psychiatry (in press)

Kiivet RA, Llerena A, Dahl ML, Rootslane L, Sanchez Vega J, Eklundh T, Sjoqvist F (1995) Patterns of drug treatment of schizophrenic patients in Estonia, Spain and Sweden. Br J Clin Pharmacol 40: 467–476

Kramer MS, Last B, Getson A, Reines SA (1997) The effects of a selective D4 dopamine receptor antagonist (L 745.870) in acutely psychotic inpatients with schizophrenia. Arch Gen Psychiatry 54: 567–572

Kulkarni J, de Castella A, Smith D, Taffe J, Keks N, Copolov D (1996) A clinical trial of the effects of estrogen in acutely psychotic women. Schizophr Res 20: 247–252

Kulkarni J, Riedel A, de Castella AR, Fitzgerald PB, Rolfe TJ, Taffe J, Burger H (2002) A clinical trial of adjunctive oestrogen treatment in women with schizophrenia. Arch Women Ment Health 5: 99–104

Lindamer LA, Buse DC, Lohr JB, Jeste DV (2001) Hormone replacement therapy in postmenopausal women with schizophrenia: positive effect on negative symptoms? Biol Psychiatry 49: 47–51

Lingjaerde O (1991) Benzodiazepines in the treatment of schizophrenia: an update survey. Acta Psychiatr Scand 84: 453–459

Mahadik SP, Evans D, Lal H (2001) Oxidative stress and role of antioxidant and omega-3 essential fatty acid supplementation in schizophrenia. Prog Neuropsychopharmacol Biol Psychiatry 25: 463–493

Marder SR, Davis JM, Chouinard G (1997) The effects of risperidone on the five dimensions of schizophrenia derived by factor analysis: combined results of the North American trials. J Clin Psychiatry 58: 538–546

McGavin JK, Goa KL (2002) Aripiprazole. CNS Drugs 16: 779–786

Muller MJ, Wetzel H, Eich FX, Rein W, Puech A, Benkert O, Amisulpride Study Group (2002) Dose-related effects of amisulpride on five dimensions of psychopathology in patients with acute exacerbation of schizophrenia. J Clin Psychopharmacol 22: 554–560

Pappadopulos E, Jensen PS, Schur SB, MacIntyre JC, Ketner S, Van Ordem K, Sverd J, Sardana S, Woodlock D, Schweitzer R, Rube D (2002) "Real world" atypical antipsychotic prescribing practices in public child and adolescent inpatient settings. Schizophr Bull 28: 111–121

Peet M, Brind J, Ramchand CN, Shah S, Vankar GK (2001) Two double-blind placebo-controlled pilot studies of eicosapentaenoic acid in the treatment of schizophrenia. Schizophr Res 49: 243–251

Peet M, Horrobin DF, E-E Multicentre Study Group (2002) A dose-ranging exploratory study of the effects of ethyl-eicosapentaenoate in patients with persistent schizophrenic symptoms. J Psychiatr Res 36: 7–18

Peuskens J, Van Baelen B, De Smedt C, Lemmens P (2000) Effects of risperidone on affective symptoms in patients with schizophrenia. Int Clin Psychopharmacol 15: 343–349

Peuskens J, Moller HJ, Puech A (2002) Amisulpride improves depressive symptoms in acute exacerbations of schizophrenia: comparison with haloperidol and risperidone. Eur Neuropsychopharmacol 12: 305–310

Potkin SG, Jin Y, Bunney BG, Costa J, Gulasekaram B (1999) Effect of clozapine and adjunctive high-dose glycine in treatment-resistant schizophrenia. Am J Psychiatry 156: 145–147
Riecher-Roessler A (2002) Oestrogen effects in schizophrenia and their potential therapeutic implications. Arch Women Ment Health 5: 111–118
Riecher-Roessler A, Häfner H, Stumbaum M, Schmidt R (1994) Do estrogens have an antipsychotic action? Fortschr Neurol Psychiatr 62: 22–28
Rittmannsberger H, Meise U, Schauflinger K, Horvath E, Donat H, Hinterhuber H (1999) Polypharmacy in psychiatric treatment. Patterns of psychotropic drug use in Austrian psychiatric clinics. Eur Psychiatry 14: 33–30
Rowley H, Kilpatrick I, Needham P, Heal D (1998) Elevation of extracellular cortical norardrenaline may contribute to the antidepressant activity of zotepine: an in vivo microdialysis study in freely moving rats. Neuropharmacol 37: 937–944
Sartorius N, Fleischhacker WW, Gjerris A, Kern U, Knapp M, Leonard BE, Lieberman JA, Lopez-Ibor JJ, van Raay B, Twomey E (2002) The usefulness and use of second-generation antipsychotic mediation. Curr Opin Psychiatry 15 [Suppl 1]: S1-S51
Schulz SC, Thompson PA, Jacobs M, Ninan PT, Robinson D, Weiden PJ, Yadalam K, Glick ID, Odbert CL (1999) Lithium augmentation fails to reduce symptoms in poorly responsive schizophrenic outpatients. J Clin Psychiatry 60: 366–72
See RE (2000) The role of neurotransmitter receptors in the adverse effects of antipsychotic drugs. In: Lidow MS (ed) Neurotransmitter receptors in actions of antipsychotic medication. CRC Press, Boca Raton London New York Washington DC, pp 221–242
Shiloh R, Zemishlany Z, Aizenberg D, Radwan M, Schwartz B, Dorfman-Etrog P, Modai I, Khaikin M, Weizman A (1997) Sulpiride augmentation in people with schizophrenia partially responsive to clozapine. A double-blind, placebo-controlled study. Br J Psychiatry 171: 569–573
Tandon R, Harrigan E, Zorn SH (1997) Ziprasidone: a novel antipsychotic with unique pharmacology and therapeutic potential. J Serotonin Res 4: 159–177
Tollefson GD, Sanger TM, Beasley CM, Tran PV (1998) A double-blind, controlled comparison of the novel antipsychotic olanzapine versus haloperidol or placebo on anxious and depressive symptoms accompanying schizophrenia. Biol Psychiatry 43: 803–810
Ungvari GS, Kau LS, Wai-Kwong T, Shing NF (2001) The pharmacological treatment of catatonia: an overview. Eur Arch Psychiatry Clin Neurosci 251 [Suppl 1]: I31–34
Wassef AA, Dott SG, Harris A, Brown A, O'Boyle M, Meyer WJ 3rd, Rose RM (1999) Critical review of GABA-ergic drugs in the treatment of schizophrenia. J Clin Psychopharmacol 19: 222–232
Wolkowitz OM, Pickar D (1991) Benzodiazepines in the treatment of schizophrenia: a review and reappraisal. Am J Psychiatry 148: 714–726
Wright P, Birkett M, David SR, Meehan K, Ferchland I, Alaka KJ, Saunders JC, Krueger J, Bradley P, San L, Bernardo M, Reinstein M, Breier A (2001) Double-blind, placebo-controlled comparison of intramuscular olanzapine and intramuscular haloperidol in the treatment of acute agitation in schizophrenia. Am J Psychiatry 158: 1149–1151

Author's address: W. W. Fleischhacker, MD, Department of Biological Psychiatry, Innsbruck University Clinics, Anichstrasse 35, A-6020 Innsbruck, Austria, e-mail: wolfgang.fleischhacker@uibk.ac.at

Springer-Verlag
and the Environment

GPSR Compliance

The European Union's (EU) General Product Safety Regulation (GPSR) is a set of rules that requires consumer products to be safe and our obligations to ensure this.

If you have any concerns about our products, you can contact us on ProductSafety@springernature.com

In case Publisher is established outside the EU, the EU authorized representative is:

Springer Nature Customer Service Center GmbH
Europaplatz 3
69115 Heidelberg, Germany

Batch number: 10578403

Printed by Printforce, the Netherlands